The Rigl

For families and

The Right To The Truth

For families and friends of patients with cancer

By I. C. PAPACHRISTOS, M.D.

English edition edited by George A. Rossetti

With a Foreword by Peter Goldstraw

www.papachristos.eu/righttothetruth

Book translated into English by the author with the assistance of George A. Rossetti:

www.papachristos.eu/righttothetruth

Book first published in Greek on June 26, 2016 (Greek book's ISBN 978-960-93-8208-3): www.papachristos.eu/dsa

ISBN 978-1977834744

*To **the memory** of my beloved mother **Panagiota** (1930–2004), the Red Cross volunteer nurse who bestowed me with the blessing of Life, and to her father, **Dr. Ioannis A. Princephiles** (1885–1956), and to **all souls** who provided "for the benefit of the sick."*

*And ye shall know **the truth**, and*

the truth *shall make you free*

John 8:32 (King James Bible)

Table of Contents

A Foreword by Peter Goldstraw

In the last 50 years the investigation and management of cancer has been a major part of my professional life. In the late 1960s many patients were content to be told that the doctor recommended this test or this treatment, often ignoring or pushing away offers of further information as to why such treatment was necessary or what alternatives were available. As a junior doctor working over 100 hours a week such unquestioning faith was flattering and time-saving, but as one gained experience and seniority one came to appreciate the overwhelming responsibility one assumed in such a parent–child–like relationship.

The situation was even more fraught when dealing with patients whose knowledge of English was poor, and one often suspected that the translator did not pass on all of the information one had intended to give to the patient and their relatives.

Fortunately, in most developed countries, the legislative framework and ethical environment have long since changed the doctor-patient relationship, and not just in cancer management. These changes have been largely led by patients and their families, and welcomed by all of the health care professionals involved in the patient's journey. Information and advice is now sought by the patient, their families and advocates from the primary care physician, every member of the hospital specialist team, and latterly the internet. It has become widely recognised that no patient can give "informed consent" for investigation or treatment unless they are fully aware of their diagnosis, the extent and severity of the condition, the impact of pre-existing diagnoses, and the risks and benefit of all options for investigation and treatment.

Imparting "bad news" requires training and takes time. The patient often hears nothing more once the word "cancer" has been spoken and the information provided has to be kept to digestible amounts, often repeated, and tailored to each person's capacity to absorb. How else can a patient make a decision to proceed with treatment, often at great expense, that disrupts their professional and family life, requires hospital time, is associated with unpleasant and painful side effects, and may entail a risk to life, when they have no real appreciation of the possible benefit they may gain? Providing the patient with all of the information necessary for them to give informed consent often allows appropriate "good news" to be given, providing hope in a dark situation.

Dr. Ioannis Papachristos spent some years of his training in a health care system where a culture of openness was practiced and has since continued his practice within an environment in which the old paternalistic approach of "protecting" the patient from the truth of their condition is still common.

He has seen how the latter approach frequently does not deceive the patient, who is deep down aware that such invasive tests and major treatment could not be justified for the benign and trivial condition from which they are told they are afflicted. If the patient is cured then other sufferers are deprived of the hope provided by such a positive outcome. Sometimes, recurrence of the disease demands further investigation and treatment, and with that more complicated deceptions. Ultimately the deception cannot be continued and the despairing patient loses all trust in their physician and even their own family. At the most taxing time in their lives, sometimes at the very end of their lives, they feel deserted and deprived of the emotional support they so desperately seek!

In this book Dr. Papachristos sets out the arguments for such an open approach, for all conditions not just cancer, and offers real and practical advice as to how such a policy can be implemented in clinical practice. His philosophy and arguments are reinforced by fictional vignettes, amalgams of real experiences in his practice. I am sure that patients, their friends and relatives, and eventually their health care providers, will benefit from the study of this excellent book. Through my own experience I can assure them that they will come to appreciate that such an open approach to the truth benefits not only the patient, but relieves the family, their friends, and most of all their physicians, of the burden of deception.

Peter Goldstraw,

Honorary Consultant in Thoracic Surgery, Royal Brompton Hospital, London.

Emeritus Professor of Thoracic Surgery, Imperial College, London.

Past President, the International Association for the Study of Lung Cancer, Aurora, Colorado.

Preface

A patient's fundamental, inalienable right to know the true status of his or her condition ought to be carved in stone all over the world. Indeed, the importance of this right is recognized as being so significant that it has at last been codified in legally binding texts such as the UNESCO Universal Declaration on Bioethics and Human Rights (ratified in Paris in 2005) and the Council of Europe's 1997 Convention for the Protection of Human Rights and Dignity of the Human Being with regard to the Application of Biology and Medicine.

Although patients' rights are legally protected worldwide, occasional violations continue to occur. Incidents in which cancer patients are not informed of their diagnosis take place everywhere, from the world's great cities, metropolitan areas, and capitals, to remote rural enclaves in Europe, Asia, Africa, the Americas, Australia and beyond (e.g. inhabited non–continental island states, wherever medicine is practiced).

Many arguments are offered to justify withholding bad news from patients. One example is that it's just too time consuming. A diagnosis of cancer can be, and frequently is, overwhelming; patients understandably feel shocked, stunned, terrified, perhaps desperate the moment they hear the bad news. Accordingly, during initial disclosure, patients need ample encouragement and psychological support, and that does take a lot of time. They also need answers. When patients are first informed of a cancer diagnosis, they have a lot of questions for the physician. One question leads to another, and the answers can provoke ever–more problematic questions that a physician might not even be able to answer honestly without additional testing, but the patient needs all the answers now. There is no denying that disclosing a cancer diagnosis is an emotionally charged, time-consuming event.

It should come as no surprise, then, that some physicians choose to withhold the diagnosis and not inform their patients that they have a malignant disease. Physicians who willfully choose to mislead their patients like this are obliged to find plausible reasons to justify this unscrupulous policy. Some cynically claim they shield their patients from the truth out of compassion; it's the right thing to do because patients must be spared from the distress an unpleasant diagnosis might provoke. In fact, some older-generation physicians may genuinely believe it is their duty to withhold bad news from their patients. There was a time when this was considered, not only acceptable behavior, but the compassionate thing to do. They are products of an earlier era; the consensus today, as affirmed by the UNESCO Declaration and the Council of Europe's 1997 Convention, is that physicians are duty-bound to inform their patients of their diagnosis.

Apart from the inordinate amount of time breaking bad news requires (from the physician's perspective), disclosure is abandoned or aborted in the majority of cases because of difficulty and tension experienced by the physicians during previous patient encounters. They are so unnerved and haunted by past experiences with disclosing bad news that they can't face it again and choose instead to avoid entirely this inherently painful responsibility. Or, some physicians say they "decide whether or not to carry through with disclosure" based on their careful assessment of how the patient reacts as he gradually broaches the subject. These physicians will say they "attempted" to disclose, yet "had to abandon" the process as soon as they saw the patient's growing distress. Since it is the rare patient indeed who reacts with mounting joy while learning he has cancer, these physicians, in effect, never follow through with disclosure, though some (out of embarrassment) might claim they inform "a few."

In more sinister (and one hopes fewer) cases, nondisclosure is systematically and routinely practiced with malevolent ulterior motives in mind, with the aim of deceiving emotionally vulnerable patients and their families by *exploiting false hopes* for profit, as will be exposed below.

Patients' families are often placed in the difficult position of having to decide whether or not to disclose a diagnosis of cancer to their loved ones. It is a dilemma that few are prepared for, and they tend to make decisions based on raw emotions alone rather than reason. These families need to be taught how to think things through calmly and rationally, so they can make reasoned choices about what is best for the well-being of their loved ones, especially when called upon to make decisions that might deeply strain them emotionally.

This book attempts to offer supportive advice for families, for patients, and for all professionals involved in the care of cancer patients. This book offers a wealth of arguments in favor of respecting and ensuring patients' right to know the truth. These arguments are framed in the context of clinical case studies that end very badly for patients because a diagnosis was withheld or because the patient was lied to. In addition, this book describes in great detail a structured, systematic method for breaking bad news to patients; attending physicians might find that some of the ideas offered complement their own personal style of providing information. Finally, this book is a clarion call for truth in all aspects of the doctor–patient relationship.

Truth in medicine, of course, extends far beyond disclosing a diagnosis. Patients are entitled to know the nature and characteristics of their disease, the factors involved in staging, and the risks and benefits associated with available, indicated treatments. Above all, they must understand the prognosis associated with treatment "A" versus treatment "B" versus no treatment at all. A patient's signed consent to proceed with a given treatment is valid only when he or she understands fully the pros and cons of all available choices. Unfortunately, too many patients agree to undergo therapies they do not fully understand, because they were not adequately informed or, all too often, intentionally deceived or coerced to sign a consent form.

A CNN article* published in June 2017 shows that, even in the United States, patients are far too often unaware of the true nature—curative, palliative, even experimental—of treatments they undergo for cancer or are left unaware of key elements of their condition. The reasons for this are many and complex; physicians overestimate their patients' knowledge about their condition, patients and physicians don't always communicate effectively, and so on. But there are cases where physicians simply withhold information patients need to plan ahead, or they intentionally provide patients with exaggerated survival times. The latter robs patients of the ability to plan realistically for the future.

Patients are also at risk of being deceived and manipulated for profit. In wealthy, developed countries, such as the US, with a predominantly private health-care system, as well as in countries with a substantial private sector that coexists with a "national" or state-owned health service, the questionable motives, tempting opportunities, and financial incentives of the many stakeholders involved in cancer care (from individual practitioners to industry giants)

---

* "Despite options, many cancer patients are left in the dark," on June
15, 2017:
http://edition.cnn.com/2017/06/15/health/cancer-patients-answers-partner/

are all cause for great concern. Thus, patients need to be protected from exploitation or abuse by being fully informed.

I strongly believe that every facet of the wide array of issues relevant to cancer patients and their families should be disclosed and thoroughly explained to protect them from those who would take advantage of the vulnerable for profit. Toward this end, patient aptitude must be taken into consideration. Facts and findings should be described clearly in *terms a given patient can understand;* they must be able to comprehend what they hear. An ignorant patient is a vulnerable patient; and predatory physicians do, sadly, exist.

Unfortunately, bad things do happen where you might least expect it. In Britain, for example, a 59-year-old surgeon* was sentenced to prison after being convicted of "wounding with intent" nine women and one man. According to an article that appeared in *The Mirror*, he

---

* "Sick surgeon who butchered breast cancer patients and performed unnecessary ops is struck off" on The Mirror, July 25, 2017: http://www.mirror.co.uk/news/uk-news/sick-surgeon-who-butchered-breast-10870306#ICID=sharebar_facebook

"butchered" cancer patients, performed unnecessary operations, and he exploited vulnerable patients for his own gain by charging for these surgical procedures. These things do happen, albeit rarely. Still, some of my colleagues in the greater medical community routinely make bad choices; sometimes for the sake of convenience and sometimes out of personal greed. Whatever the reason, it is the patient who suffers in the end.

In this book, readers will find stories, at once interesting and appalling, of patients who suffered terribly, and unnecessarily, because they were deliberately deceived by their physicians. Case studies are provided of actual incidents that I have witnessed or otherwise have personal knowledge of. These stories, which appear at the beginning of each chapter, are called "*Clinical Counterexamples*." The stories are inspired by—or based on—true events, but the names have been changed to protect the privacy of all persons involved. It is hoped that the lessons learned from these Counterexamples will serve to raise awareness among patients and health–care professionals alike, and that steps will be taken to ensure that patients no longer suffer the consequences of being denied the truth. My sole purpose for writing "The Right To The Truth" is to promote the protection of, and respect for, patients' rights; it is in no way intended to raise pointless accusations against any person or provoke senseless scandals.

It's hardly a secret that we live in an imperfect world. Bad things happen to good people. It's bad enough that some of them get cancer; what's even worse is that the very people they look to for treatment, support, and hope would lie to them, withhold information they need, or even exploit them for profit. We must, all of us, appeal to the "better angels of our nature" and try to make it a better world for cancer patients by simply telling them the truth and showing sincere compassion and empathy. Let us stand by them as trusted allies, offering all the support they so badly need as they fight their disease.

Prologue of the Greek, original edition

This book was written for the purpose of offering support, advice, and compassion *to the families and friends* of cancer patients. In many countries populated by peoples known for their openly emotional and compassionate natures, such as those in the Mediterranean regions, patients are often left unaware of their own diagnosis of cancer, or other similarly serious disease!

If readers find it difficult to believe this still happens today, in the 21st century, they need look no further than what has become common, everyday practice in Greece. Unfortunate, ordinary people suddenly find themselves in the awkward position of facing the dilemma of whether or not to let their close relative know they've been diagnosed with a serious disease. This dilemma, however, was never meant to be theirs to face. For they were not trained how to break bad news, they lack professional experience in this area, and they should never have been informed of the diagnosis in the first place!

Respect, hope, truth, and compassion are what this book attempts to provide *to patients* as well, should they decide to read it. They need to know the truth if they are to fight a serious disease and make informed decisions about treatment options.

The treatment options recommended usually carry risks of side effects, but they are also associated with promising possibilities—not certainties—of favorable outcomes or even cures. Considering, pondering and weighing treatment options is already a full-time job for patients. It requires their thorough attention and thoughtful deliberation as it is, so they are at a distinct disadvantage if clinical factors are obscured by lies, false promises, and diagnoses withheld or kept secret.

Throughout the entire 32 years this author has been involved in practicing medicine, he has always been frustrated by the *disgrace* that continuously occurs in Greece all the time. The author has been hurt by this contemporary equivalent of the ancient *"Cylonian affair"* * curse.

---

* The sacrilegious execution of Suppliants in front of goddess Athena's Temple on the Acropolis in 632 BC (by the clan of Alcmaeonidae). The Suppliants originated from the

Patients nowadays are routinely informed of cancer diagnoses even in countries where this wasn't always the case in the past, such as in Portugal, Turkey, and Colombia! Of course, for many decades patients have been, and continue to be, informed of their diagnoses and provided with accurate details in developed countries, such as the United States, Britain, Germany, and others. Yet, in the birthplace of Hippocrates, a culture that fosters patient unawareness has become so deeply entrenched in the everyday practice of medicine that it seems not to bother anyone. In fact, it might even suit some depraved, unrighteous, and wicked persons.

Patients are regularly kept in the darkness of ignorance and puzzlement regarding their condition. Even worse, they are at risk of being exploited by cunning

---

city–state of Megara and were led by Cylon. They had unsuccessfully attempted seizure of power (a coup) in Athens; then they took refuge in the Temple of "Polias Athena" (a sacred and inviolable asylum). The ancient Athenians thought that the infamous execution was to blame (as a moral taint) for the subsequent epidemics, bad crops, and other disasters (then considered acts of gods) that struck their city–state. "Cylonian affair" is forever synonymous with the disgrace or shame of a state or country.

professionals who may be motivated by the prospect of profiting in some nefarious way by instilling false hope.

Patients eventually do learn the truth, however, as their disease progresses. Or, sooner or later, something else happens that leads to disclosure; then, these patients have lost any confidence—justifiably so—in their own families or in the medical profession in general. If this occurs, then such a patient has no one to turn to (or, to quote scripture, "man hath not where to lay his head" *) during the most difficult, sacred moments of his or her life. Such a thing is definitely cruel and inhumane!

This book seeks to eliminate the contemporary taint, to shed ample light on the darkness of hypocrisy and unawareness, to promote truthfulness, and to soothe human sorrow. It also attempts to heal a *festering wound* in our land; this national wound invites sharp-taloned ravens to encircle sufferers for pecuniary interests of their own. This book tries *to strike a blow*, to awaken consciousness, to improve things "for the benefit of the sick" † .

Reason and common sense is what this book attempts to provide *to physicians;* ie, to the author's

---

* Matthew 8:20 (King James's bible)
† Quote from the Hippocratic Oath: " ἐπ' ὠφελείῃ καμνόντων "

colleagues. They need to remember that Hippocrates taught us the primacy of the patient above all else as well as *empathy* and compassion and to always stand beside the patient.

There can be no bond between physician and patient without mutual respect and trust, which can only be built on the solid ground of truth. If I respect my patients as their doctor, then I tell them the truth, because it is their right to know. Patient-physician confidentiality forbids me from informing anyone else other than the patient. It is up to the patients to decide whether or not they want to disclose their diagnosis to family and friends. In any given case of a family facing the dilemma of whether or not to inform the patient of a diagnosis, a physician has been guilty of breaching his or her obligation for confidentiality. Families should never be placed in such a situation in the first place!

The majority of physicians, of course, have the best of intentions and always mean well, yet some of them should have a better sense of their obligations. They are expected to act as professionals; physicians cannot pretend to be unaware of their own obligations to let their patients know first. It is simply preposterous for anyone to claim ignorance of this!

Doctors are also expected to be competent in their bedside manners, to express empathy or compassion for their patients, to support them, and to know how—as professionals—to break bad news to them. Physicians are not only supposed to be awarded by fees or praise for favorable outcomes; they are also expected to be there, present, standing beside their patients for good or for worse, offering humane support, or else deep learning algorithms and similar software will soon replace them for good!

This book also endeavors to provide *the unsung heroes*—nurses, physiotherapists, lab technicians, paramedics, and support staff—with helpful material for their consideration. This will aid them in the fight against obscurantism, hypocrisy, and ignorance.

Nursing staff is the cornerstone of the whole system of practicing modern medicine. It is from the nurses' hands that a glass of water will be offered to patients in order to refresh their dry mouth; it is from the nurses' hands that pain killers and other medications will be given for easing suffering; it is also from the very same hands that chemotherapy and other intravenous medication will be administered. Patients need to trust whatever is offered by those competent, experienced, overworked hands on the solid basis of truth.

Finally, it is the nurses whom patients speak with directly, easily, and often after admission into a hospital. Nurses' truthful attitudes can be a balm to patients' souls. Nursing staffs are sacred allies of the medical fight against cancer!

There will be some benefit from reading this book even *for those who happen to adopt the opposite opinion* (for those who favor the patients' unawareness of their own cancer diagnosis). One becomes wiser by also considering the "altera pars" (the arguments and counterexamples in this book) or by considering various viewpoints while examining a subject.

The author's rationale* and clinical experience are illustrated with clarity and enthusiasm; they result in practical instruction for how patients should be better informed. This may be considered an enduring contribution, for it is an opinion now recorded in the literature. From now on it will

---

* The term "rationale" means that an explanation or justification is given for each thought / statement. The thoughts presented are "not unsubstantiated," but they rely on some kind of justification.

always be accessible to any clinician, any caregiver for patients, any "res cogitans" *.

The "polytonic" spelling (with accents, "iota underlined" etc.) is consistently maintained throughout this book for Hellenic (ancient Greek) words in phrases, such as the ones quoted by Hippocrates (e.g., " ἐπ' ὠφελείῃ καμνόν-των " meaning "for the benefit of the sick"). The very same spelling is also maintained for all words that have remained unchanged in everyday common speech of modern Greek after having travelled through time for a few millennia.

There now exists a modern, innovative way of presenting author's notes in the *ePub* (electronic publication) version of this book. These occur in the form of interactive author's notes instead of conventional footnotes: when readers press on the two underlined symbols ⬇️📭 on the surface of the tablet (iPad or similar) or when they mouse click on them, a yellow box containing the note pops up. When the reader clicks outside the yellow box it closes, allowing the reader to carry on with the main text. In future print versions of the same book, author's notes will, of course, appear as conventional footnotes.

---

* Res cogitans: Latin term for a "thinking / contemplating individual" in philosophy

Nearly every chapter of the book begins with a *clinical counterexample* inspired by the author's 32 years' clinical experience: the tribulations and catastrophes described in each counterexample show eloquently, cynically, sorely, and practically how invariably disastrous it is when patients are denied knowledge of their own true diagnosis.

No counterexample represents an actual event or fact. Any resemblance to real persons is purely coincidental. The whole duration of thirty two years gets contracted in order to be accommodated into few pages full of counterexamples and it gets dilated for the author to be able to answer to the question: " doctor, what do you see and observe throughout your whole life health–wise ? "

Real persons may have inspired some of the characters or situations dramatized in some of the counterexamples, but they have no association with the stories themselves whatsoever. Names of people and places used are fictitious. The author has cause to worry that reality may actually be far worse in Greece than the clinical counterexamples herein suggest.

1.

In the Limelight of Imperial Capitals And Out of It

Historic Fact

The guards and everyone else in Buckingham Palace were puzzled by the presence of a peculiar scent—that of iodine and other antiseptic agents—permeating the air of the first floor in September of 1951. The strange odors wafted from freshly opened containers in the Buhl room, which had been converted into an operating theatre. In that room on September 23, His Majesty King George VI underwent major surgery wherein his left lung was removed because of cancer. The left recurrent laryngeal nerve also had to be removed during the procedure, which subsequently caused the King to speak with a hoarse voice.

His Majesty was completely unaware that he had cancer, despite his thoracic surgeon's intention to be frank. The surgeon, Sir Clement Price Thomas, was overruled by higher authorities. Thus, the unfortunate sovereign was deprived of the same patients' rights already enjoyed by all his subjects during that era. The diagnosis was withheld from the noblest patient in the realm to benefit the interests of the mighty Empire that was soon to be reduced to a Kingdom. A few months after surgery, King George was finally informed of the truth about his cancer, when disease recurrence made further deception impossible.

Continuation of Chapter 1

Unfortunately, occasional violations of a patient's basic right to know the true status of their own condition do take place throughout the world. Of course, "the greater good" is invariably held forth in defense of such inhumane violations of trust; sometimes for the ostensible benefit of the patient or, as is more often the case, for the benefit of others surrounding the patient. In some cultures, nondisclosure by physicians is almost customary and justified as a courtesy to the patient, as in Japan for instance, where informing patients they have cancer might be regarded as a cruel or unkind act!

In far distant places and countries around the globe inhabited by people known for their passionate or highly emotional natures (e.g., Mediterranean countries), a family member may well demand withholding a difficult-to-reveal diagnosis from a loved one. In Portugal, Turkey, Latin America and elsewhere some relatives are tormented as they weigh the pros and the cons of letting their loved one know they have a frightening diagnosis.

One may think that it is only in rural places and among the peasantry as well as in deserts of the Arabian Peninsula and in remote areas of countries such as Iran, Qatar,

Egypt, etc. where patients are kept uninformed by illiterate relatives. Nondisclosure, however, routinely takes place even in urbane, civilized cities and capitals in Europe and elsewhere. Even inside imperial palaces, as we know. Excessive, but ultimately unwise, concerns about a patient's emotional state may lead to the extreme of withholding the diagnosis altogether, as happens in some cases in France or Italy.

From the physician's perspective, breaking bad news to patients is often difficult and unpleasant. Many physicians the world over are discomfited by the emotional burden of having to reveal unpleasant truths to their patients. Hence, some young or inexperienced physicians may opt for the gambit of delaying disclosure, thus buying time—they hope—for information to be provided to the patient by some relative or by any other person willing to do so. The problem with this, of course, is that untrained nonprofessionals are likely unqualified for the task at hand and might resort to amateurish improvisations, which won't benefit the patient at all. Perpetual delaying of disclosure may lead to complete unawareness wholesale!

Patients intentionally left in the dark about their own cancer diagnosis are found all over the world. Yet no other country on Earth is as unique in this context as Greece, where patient unawareness is rampant. In Greece, the great majority of physicians refrain from informing their patients of their true diagnosis in order, ostensibly, to "spare them any distress." It is estimated that as many as approximately 79% of Greek physicians have never told even one patient about his / her cancer diagnosis during the entirety of their professional lives! Even if the actual percentage of those who do so is somehow lower, the clinical practice of withholding cancer diagnoses is exceedingly widespread in Greece.

Thus, Greece will serve as a model in this book. Clinical stories involving unaware patients, as the reader will see, reveal how withholding information inevitably led to major catastrophes that ought to be inconceivable in the modern era. These stories herein will be called "*counterexamples*." Each clinical story—inspired by true events from the author's medical experience—will stimulate critical thinking and arguments about what is best "for the benefit of the sick," as Hippocratic ethics demand.

Whenever in Japan, or Lebanon, or even the UK, one even considers hiding the cancer diagnosis from a relative (or from one's patient), then one might learn valuable lessons by reading about the consequences of other people's mistakes caused by depriving patients of their inalienable right to know the truth!

2.

When Bad News Breaks

Clinical Counterexample

For several months, Magdalene had been suffering from gastrointestinal discomfort and irregular bowel movements, with alternating episodes of constipation and diarrhea. After noticing blood in her stool, she grew quite concerned and made an appointment for a return visit to her gastroenterologist.

She was a kind-hearted, middle-aged widow, mother, and caregiver to her young daughter, who suffered from a rare autoimmune disease. Magdalene's husband had recently died of a sudden heart attack. In light of the stress associated with caring for a dependent child and profound grief over the unexpected loss of her husband, Magdalene's gastroenterologist initially diagnosed her complaints as symptoms of a psychomotor disorder or possibly attributable to a mild form of colitis. The presence of occult fecal blood, however, warranted an endoscopy. Analysis of biopsy specimens obtained during the procedure confirmed a diagnosis of colon cancer.

The diagnosis greatly distressed Magdalene's brother and young daughter. They were uncertain how to tell her the truth about her condition, or whether she should be told at all. How much more bad news can a grieving new widow, already at her wits' end, possibly handle? Especially one responsible for the care and well-being of a sick child? Magdalene's daughter and brother—the only surviving members of her family—were consumed with despair and profoundly anxious over how to handle the news.

Continuation of Chapter 2

If you have learned that a close family member of yours suffers from cancer (or any serious, life-threatening disease) please don't despair! Be strong! Cancer is indeed a scary diagnosis, but great advances in medical science mean that hope in our era is well founded and warranted.

You'll probably wonder why cause for such *hope* exists. Well, in your own loved one's case—*depending on disease stage and cancer cell type*—one might reasonably hope for a cure. You did not misread—cure might be possible, or extension of survival time and improvement in quality of life, or at least palliation of symptoms (improvement in quality of life and pain relief during their remaining days). All cause for hope is grounded in documented positive outcomes achieved using existing methods of treating cancer. That is to say, current-day, clinically tested treatment methods offer considerable potential for cure in many cases and more favorable outcomes in general.

For example, cure rates in cases of stage p**I**a NSCLC (non-small cell lung cancer), are as high as 73%. Moreover, hope for cure exceeds this percentage in early stage disease and cancers that are less aggressive biologically than lung cancer. In testicular cancer, for example, cure rates of 90% to 95% are reported if disease is diagnosed early enough and treated appropriately. In stage I testicular cancer, the cure rate exceeds 98%.

So, a family member who has just received bad news should be encouraged to remain calm, to try to relax, and to consider that a diagnosis of cancer isn't necessarily as hopeless as was once widely thought. Of course, it remains unpleasant and frightening, but cancer is manageable by contemporary medicine. Today, therapeutic measures and strategies exist that can be applied to treat and offer improvement to almost all patients. The first fact one should bear in mind after being diagnosed with any malignant disease is that it is not necessarily the end of the world. Therapeutic help exists and will be offered. Again, there truly is cause for hope!

The second fact one needs to be reminded of is how deleterious some practices have been for our society as a whole. Traditionally, past practices have always been full of negative connotations such as use of the term "~~Loathsome~~

disease" (for cancer in modern Greek*) and the practice of withholding the true diagnosis from the very party who is directly involved and affected.

Close family members have also been withholding the diagnosis from the patients' wider social sphere (colleagues, neighbors, non-immediate family members) to prevent accidental disclosure to the patient. Consequently, our society has been encouraged—and continuously so for decades—to face cancer in an unhealthy, counterproductive way. The good news that patients are being cured of cancer isn't getting out to the public; they hear only the worst possible news. Because news of cancer diagnoses has been systematically suppressed, the general population in Greece is largely unaware that patients were and are being cured. Cause for celebration exists, but an oblivious population doesn't know that. Consequently, they've been deprived of the opportunity to celebrate and applaud advances in oncology and share in the happiness of health restored to persons with cancer.

Modern Greek society, kept in the dark about advances in cancer treatment and increasing cases of

---

* In Greek, the actual term is: "η ~~Επάρατη~~ νόσος," pronounced "ee Eparati nossos."

patients cured, learn only of the most unpleasant outcomes. Bad news often arrives through social media and obituaries in newspapers about patients who succumbed to cancer. That the numbers of such patients has dwindled significantly—the good news—isn't being reported. Thus, society has unfortunately and continuously been groomed *a priori* to consider the final outcome as predetermined— sadness and sorrow for each and every new patient diagnosed with cancer. All their lives residents of small towns heard news about funerals of people who died of cancer, yet these very same people remained unaware that survivors today may well twice outnumber the deceased. If people only knew how many others around us defeated cancer in the past, there would be far less fear of this disease today. We would live in a better informed, happier world; a world free of unnecessary, unwarranted fear.

All these unknown patients, those who survived their disease, were treated with conventional existing therapies. All the more astonishing is that many of these survivors, people who live and work among us every day, are themselves completely unaware that they ever had cancer. I cannot possibly emphasize this fact enough, because even more reason for hope will be presented in the text that follows.

As this book is being written, scientific research carries on, spectacular progress takes place, new data come to light, and innovative ways to treat cancer are being tested, including studies employing immunotherapy, vaccines, targeted methods based on genes and nanoparticles, to name a few promising areas. Battles are being won and more therapeutic knowledge is acquired daily.

Unpredictable leaps of progress have occurred many times in the history of medicine. The serendipitous discovery of penicillin by Sir Alexander Fleming in 1928, for example, as well as subsequent, and ongoing, discovery of other antibiotics can only feed us with expectations and well-founded hope.

Unprecedented efforts and resources are being invested in the fight against cancer. Multinational corporations involved in pharmaceutical development, diagnostics, imaging, medical device design and manufacture, and all manner of tools and technology necessary to understand and defeat cancer are daily pouring untold billions into research and development. It is truly a battle of epic proportions waged by a cooperative international community of experts determined to win.

The only possible outcome of this monumental campaign is that the destructive force of cancer will be mastered by humanity's stubborn commitment to do the "impossible," just as the flow of the Chicago river was reversed in 1900 (the river now flows out from Lake Michigan instead of into it), and the Panama Canal divided the American continent in two halves, etc. Cancer will be defeated with the same determination it required to conquer space, because the stakes are even higher.

Failure is inconceivable. Too much time, money, and tenacious human resolve have been invested in the war on cancer. Day after day we get ever nearer to finding the answers we need. This solution may astonish all in the end if it materializes with suddenness, as was the case with the discoveries of potent treatments for similarly lethal diseases in the past (tuberculosis, syphilis, leprosy etc.).

And so, to all friends, family, and loved ones of patients with cancer, you now know that there's no reason for all-consuming despair. Cancer is always an unwelcome diagnosis; some forms of the disease respond well and completely to current treatments; other types can be very difficult to control. Yet, effective treatments that lead to satisfactory outcomes do exist, and even more effective methods are being developed all the time. The important point to remember is that potential for cure does exist.

The patient will definitely need your moral support, your presence through the struggle, your encouragement, someone to wipe away tears and instill hope. And you alone—a trusted family member, a close friend or relative who has known the patient for years—are the only person in the world who can provide the level of compassionate, deeply personal emotional care and spiritual sustenance the patient will need. Cancer is a disease, the patient's emotional reaction to the diagnosis is not. Accordingly, there is absolutely no need to involve psychiatrists or psychologists in the patient's care. They can't deliver what you alone can. Yet *truth* and *sincerity* are absolutely necessary for trust, support, and the expression of humane compassion. Try not to forget about the latter!

3.

Family Members Who Resort to Deception

Clinical Counterexample

Gregory retired on his pension and lived carefree and content in his cottage by the sea. He was a genial old man enjoying his remaining years as comfortably as possible. Gregory lived alone and was able to care for himself, but the ravages of old age ailed him. Along with old age come diseases like hypertension, cardiovascular problems, diabetes, arthritis, etc. Though frail, Gregory was cheerful, optimistic, and looking forward to the rest of his life in the warm company of family and friends. But things were not as they seemed.

Neither Gregory's daughter—nor anyone else—dared break some very bad news to the elderly man. Gregory didn't know that his 42-year-old son Harry suffered a sudden stroke, lost consciousness, and had been urgently admitted to a large hospital. Harry's condition was critical. Gregory's loved ones were gravely concerned that something dreadful might happen to the fragile old man if he were informed that his son lay at death's door.

A pack of lies had to be concocted to account for the sudden loss of communication between father and son. Harry, it was alleged, was away hunting, high on a remote part of the Pindos mountain range, where he couldn't be reached because there was no cell-phone service. Gregory wasn't even informed of Harry's stroke when his condition improved, and he was no longer in immediate danger. Again, the intent was to shield Gregory from any distressing news that might sadden him.

The son survived and continued to improve, but residual neurological deficits persisted. He walked with a limp and had difficulty speaking. The old father was stunned when he at last saw Harry before him, entering the cottage. Gregory's old heart was broken the moment he noticed that his son was limping and stuttering.

Gregory wasn't cheered by evidence of Harry's survival and regaining consciousness, because the old father was never informed of those improvements, let alone that Harry suffered a stroke in the first place. All he knew was the sudden shock of seeing his son incapacitated. He had been deliberately kept in the dark all along. He didn't know that his son's condition was steadily improving. Moreover, Gregory no longer believed anyone's promises that further neurological improvement was expected to occur.

Barely 24 hours after he had first seen Harry ill, Gregory fell dead on the cottage floor while shaving, right in front of his son.

The family members once again took action. They didn't allow Harry to attend his father's funeral during his recovery, despite the fact that he bore witness to his father's death with his own eyes. As his father's funeral was taking place, Harry was taken out by some of his friends. They kept him meandering about, limping aimlessly from one café to another. Their goal was to keep him occupied and distracted, that he might forget all and not be saddened by reality. As if it were possible for this 42-year-old man to purge from his memory everything that had taken place, and was taking place at that moment!

The family members were overemotional, and their actions were impulsive. They also thought themselves to be acting in the best interests of both father and son. The relatives' lies, their suppression of truth, and exaggerations stretched the limits of what could ever be permitted by solemnity, dignity, common sense, and human decency. Yet they escaped an awkward position. The tragedy was beyond their control; they themselves broke no bad news and couldn't be held responsible for the inevitable disclosure that time and nature would reveal. The latter offered sufficiently handy grounds to disavow any responsibility of their own.

In a few months' time Harry got much better and, finally, there were no residual motor or speech disorders left at all. The father, however, never took pleasure in seeing his improvement, because he was no longer there...

Continuation of Chapter 3

Erratic, grievous, distressing, sad, and disastrous events unfortunately occur whenever families choose the slippery slope of lying and withholding information, despite their undeniably good intentions. Lying can cause catastrophes even graver than the bad news itself, as was the case in the counterexample above. The old father didn't survive to enjoy seeing the full neurological recovery of his hemiplegic son. Similarly, there is hope for cure in cancer cases. It is a pity for that hope to be wasted like a storm-tossed castaway, adrift in an ocean of lies and of the patient's justifiable disbelief.

As soon as a diagnosis of cancer or similar disease is revealed to a patient's family members, they are *overwhelmed by emotions* of sorrow, grief, and despair. A subconscious self-defensive impulse called "denial" almost always gets triggered to protect them from the sudden earthquake of the distressing news. The relatives refuse to accept or believe the unbearably sad news. They harbor reservations about the diagnosis and suspect it might be incorrect. Emotions *flood* over the family members to such an extent that they become the worst guides and advisors.

Emotions impair their judgment, which makes objective reasoning impossible.

So, the relatives' usual first reactions and actions are perfectly understandable. Since they themselves disbelieve or deny the diagnosis of cancer, they naturally refuse to announce the diagnosis to the patient. They justify hiding the diagnosis under the pretext that it will only be "temporary." They plan to disclose the truth to the patient at a later moment, when at last they have accepted the diagnosis.

Yet nothing endures the temporary, especially when it is understood that revealing the diagnosis will only make things even more awkward and unbearable for themselves, regardless of how long they manage to put off. Thus, they never truly find the nerve or the "right moment" to make their relative sad or frightened by revealing such a diagnosis. They mistakenly think that they even do some good, for they are possessed by the illusion and irrational hope that grim reality will miraculously be cancelled and revoked, that it will simply be annulled or reversed, just because they hide and conceal it.

Even if the families comprehend—and few do—that the patient should know, and is entitled to know, the diagnosis and all relevant information as it pertains to his or her treatment, it is still rare that even one person among them finds the courage to proceed alone with breaking the bad news. Family members usually wait for somebody else, anybody else, perhaps a "deus ex machina," to come to the rescue and relieve them of their own difficult duty to inform. They wait in futility for a person more dispassionate or detached than themselves—perhaps a distant relative—to volunteer to break the news. Sometimes they consult psychiatrists or psychologists, as if it were schizophrenia or some other psychosis that ailed the patient, instead of cancer!

Of course, the family members are not to blame for their impulsive reactions while in the throes of indescribable grief and profound misery; they cannot help being stirred by emotions. But it makes them take erratic, inconsistent, and contradictory actions that ultimately harm the very person they hope to protect. In addition to the emotional challenges of coming to terms with bad news, confusion can also be overwhelming; few (if any) family members can be expected to understand a diagnosis, or the nature of the disease itself, or the various treatment options available. After all, few patients have relatives with degrees in health sciences or postgraduate studies. They usually lack comparative experience, too, as they generally find themselves in circumstances they're entirely unfamiliar with. So, they cannot possibly make informed, objective decisions as to what is best for the patient himself, their beloved one!

4.

Potentially Evil Intent or "Malice"

Clinical Counterexample

For many years Kieran suffered shortness of breath, even with minimal exertion, which had become increasingly debilitating over time. It reached a point where merely walking to the bathroom felt like torture, as even that modest effort left him gasping for air. He was a retired car mechanic and a long-time, heavy smoker of cigarettes. In fact, despite his breathing problems, Kieran remained a determined smoker, undeterred by his chest physician's warning that he would soon require home oxygen therapy!

So, it came as no surprise when cancer was diagnosed in his right lung. What was surprising was the decision to remove half the lung surgically. This decision was made by Eleanor, Kieran's wife. She kneeled and kissed the hands of Keefe Tousoulis, the surgeon, out of gratitude, inside a large hospital in Athens, Greece. Eleanor remained elegant and attractive in middle age, and she loved her husband Kieran; so much so that she demanded the cancer diagnosis be kept secret from him in order to "avoid causing him sadness."

The surgeon, however, had profound reservations about removing half of Kieran's lung; he was concerned about his patient's already poor respiratory function and questionable ability to survive the procedure. Plus, Kieran had a hard enough time breathing as it was, still equipped with two complete lungs.

But Kieran's wife insisted; she couldn't stand to see her beloved husband steadily deteriorating, losing weight, gradually reduced to nothing, his life slowly ebbing away as he endured protracted chemotherapy treatments. Instead, Eleanor wanted her husband to undergo surgical resection with curative intent, despite considerable risk. She understood there was a chance he could die during surgery, but if that happened he would go out, in her eyes, still looking relatively robust and strong—she would forever remember Kieran as brave and "a fit lad," as he used to be when she had fallen for him and they married, many decades ago. One couldn't help but admire Eleanor's passionate devotion to, and unerring love for, Kieran.

Results of preoperative respiratory function tests clearly revealed that pulmonary resection of any kind was absolutely contraindicated, and that Kieran was surgically unfit for the planned procedure. Yet these results would ultimately be "forgotten" by Dr. Tousoulis. After a half million drachmae were slipped to him under the table as "encouragement" to proceed with the high-risk resection, his initial reservations and clinical concerns seemingly evaporated.

The surgical goal was technically achieved. The cancer was removed by means of a lower lobectomy, and Kieran left the operating theatre alive. However, his pulmonary function, as expected, never recovered after surgery. After 11 days of mechanical ventilatory support in the Intensive Care Unit, Kieran died of respiratory failure.

Unbeknownst to all prior to Kieran's death were details surrounding an enormous amount of highly valuable property that his widow inherited in a skiing resort in central Greece.

It also came to light that for many years the grieving widow had, in fact, been quite disappointed with her husband. He suffered from severe chronic obstructive pulmonary disease (COPD), which is associated with erectile dysfunction. Kieran had indeed become impotent due to his disease, and Eleanor was angered and frustrated by the loss of intimacy in her life and her husband's inability to please her sexually. She came to think of him as a loser, especially since he was about to sign a distribution agreement with his siblings regarding inheritance. Kieran had decided to honor his father's last will (deceased in 1956), according to which he wasn't meant to be sole heir, but rather the estate property would be divided fairly and equally among all heirs. If such an agreement were signed, Eleanor felt that too little would be left for her.

Thus, the timing of her husband's death, within days of undergoing contraindicated surgery, suited Eleanor perfectly. Of course, she laid all blame at his doctors' feet; she cursed them, slandered them, and called them "murderers." Yet she managed to remain above all suspicion, untouchable, easily assuming the role of the pitiable widow. It was an amazing achievement. Eleanor would be able to manage the entirety of her late husband's estate, and do so without any emotional or moral commitments to Kieran's siblings. She would keep for herself the entire fortune, every estate, as sole heir.

Of course, no physician can be expected to have a seasoned detective's ability to foretell what true motives an ostensibly "loving wife" might have in mind when she insisted that the cancer diagnosis be withheld from her husband and then declared that she alone would assume authority to make and carry out all health care decisions for him.

Continuation of Chapter 4

Of course, no one wants to contemplate *malice** or *evil intent* as a motive of a relative who seeks to conceal a diagnosis of cancer from the patient. Yet one must always consider the possibility of an evil motive—the patient must be protected in all cases from ulterior designs, no matter how unimaginable or unthinkable they may seem. The world we live in is anything but "beautiful, moral and made by angels" † . The fiscal and financial crisis of debt in Greece and other countries at present is associated with poverty that generates nagging greed in the hearts of the wicked.

---

* "Malice" is legally defined as evil intent on the part of a person who commits a wrongful act injurious to others. "Malice aforethought" or "malice prepense" in Penal Law is a predetermination to commit an unlawful act without just cause or provocation (applied chiefly to cases of murder). Furthermore, the "dolus individualis" legal term refers to evil intent (distinguished from mere error or "culpa") making a perpetrator always liable for any damages caused.

† Quotation from the poem *"To Francesca Fraser,"* by D. Solomos (1798–1857); famous Greek poet who wrote the Hymn to Liberty: its first two stanzas became the national anthem of Greece.

For instance, a patient may well have three close relatives who simply adore him, so they want the diagnosis to remain hidden in order to spare him any anguish. This very same patient may also have another family member who may place his own interests first. Such interests may involve hereditary motives for hiding the diagnosis: to prevent the patient from changing or modifying his last will and testament at the last moment, or to prevent him from legally recognizing a natural child as his, or to prevent him from bequeathing wealth or property to an organization or favorite charity (an inalienable right of any philanthropist or religious person). Finally, the fourth relative's interests may well be to prevent the patient from undergoing any expensive treatments whose costs could make the patient's heritable fortune smaller.

Reality repeatedly proves more surprising than the most imaginative fiction writer, no matter how unfathomable the scenarios presented in the last paragraph may seem. So, the only way of assuring patients' protection is to inform them of their own diagnosis; this way the patients become empowered masters of their own decisions instead of mere prey to coveting designs of the wicked or in the lap of the gods. The attending clinician can't know the genuine motives of the patient's various relatives, nor does he possess a detective's skills. Consequently, the attending physician must provide the patient with the best guarantee of protection—truth and sincerity.

Finally, there exists the risk of cunning modern charlatans who might attempt to exploit concerned relatives' anxieties and fears by **commercializing false hopes**; i.e., by promising non-existent or fabled "magical" cures. Many of us remember notorious and painful past incidents or practices such as the infamous and fraudulent "water from Kamatero village," the "venom of the blue scorpion," as well as "heroic" attempts to perform major surgical procedures involving resection or removal of an organ, when such procedures were clinically contraindicated, due to advanced disease stage and the risk of surgery was so grave that it clearly outweighed any potential benefit.

Major surgical resections of any body part (organ) [*] should *only* be undertaken *if* and **when** clinically *indicated*, as is also the case for any medical procedure, after all. Otherwise they shouldn't be carried out. The concept of *"indication"* was conceived by Hippocrates [†].

---

[*] eg, resection of an entire lung or of the pancreas or of the liver

[†] "Those diseases which medicines do not cure, the iron cures; those which iron cannot cure, fire cures; and those which fire cannot cure are to be reckoned wholly incurable." (Hippocrates's *Aphorisms*, Section VII, 87). Meaning: the

This was the very concept that gave birth to Medicine as science, which was no longer based on subjective, arbitrary, and unsubstantiated viewpoints, as had been the case before. Hippocrates stipulated that in order to be "indicated" the benefits of any medical procedure or treatment must outweigh its risks (quotation translated into Latin as "primum non nocere"; i.e., "to help, or at least, to do no harm." Ancient Greek original quotation: "Ὠφελέειν ἢ μὴ βλάπτειν "). Since every surgical procedure carries some risk of morbidity and mortality, the anticipated benefits must outweigh those risks for the procedure to be considered "indicated."

If a patient's stage of disease is so advanced that it allows no hope at all for cure, then major surgical resection is associated with zero chance of benefit versus the considerable risks inherent in the procedure. That is to say, carrying out such surgery is contraindicated in this given

---

cauterization (with fire) of an abscess is only *indicated* to be carried out, if attempted surgical drainage of it (by a scalpel made of iron) previously failed; similarly, surgical treatment is only *indicated* after failure of previous application of medication; if all three proposed ways of treatment fail, then the disease should be considered as "incurable," i.e., there is no *indication* to apply any additional treatment method.

patient's case. If, hypothetically, he undergoes such a resection, he will be exposed to pure risk alone, bereft of any therapeutic benefit.

Furthermore, in the above hypothetical case of major surgery bearing no benefits at all, the operation will also have a profoundly adverse effect on the patient's quality of life: the procedure will force the patient to experience postoperative pain, drain(s), various catheter(s), and in-hospital stay for postoperative recovery. In such a case, the best course would have been to explain the futility and consequences of surgery, discuss palliative care, and advise the patient to enjoy his remaining life as comfortably and qualitatively as possible instead!

To be absolutely clear; on the matter of surgical removal of a tumor or resection of a human organ, one merely needs to remember that the "technical feasibility of removing a tumor" greatly differs from an "indication" to remove a tumor*. If disease stage is determined to be a

---

* For instance, removal of a tumor may well be contraindicated if there is generalized dissemination of the disease, as in cases of blood-borne spread of cancer. Surgery shouldn't just be carried out only because "it can technically" be performed; it should only be carried out when there is an indication for it. In other words, the technical feasibility

contraindication for surgical resection, then resection should not be carried out, even if some surgeon "can technically" perform it. Contraindication due to advanced disease stage always prevails and is wholly irrelevant to any surgeon's operating skill.

It is a clear case of *commercialization of false hopes* whenever a health professional promotes any clinically contraindicated "heroic" measure, such as high-risk major surgery (or any contraindicated intervention, for that matter) by promising unrealistic goals to vulnerable, highly emotional close relatives of a patient whose cancer stage is prohibitively advanced. Whenever such deceit is attempted, it is always associated with plenty of crocodile tears and supererogation designed, ostensibly, to "offer hope" to the patient. What they really offer, however, are empty promises, wishful thinking, ineffective "treatments," and risk devoid of benefit for the unfortunate patient. All benefits end up in the pockets of the wily perpetrator.

---

itself to remove a tumor is not necessarily an adequate reason for doing so; there also must be an indication for the removal of the tumor depending on its oncological stage as well as fitness of the patient to withstand and survive the operation.

It is only the patient himself who usually has the requisite instincts and intuition to feel or sense the veracity and integrity of whomever provides therapeutic advice. Accordingly, the patient must be equipped with the truth if he's to protect himself from evil intent, malice, or *dolus*... possibly by a few unscrupulous relatives, modern charlatans, or scheming experts.

5.

The Truth, Ultimately, Is Always Revealed

Clinical Counterexample

Sophie felt reassured. She was listening carefully to every word said by Associate Professor Jacob Georgiadis inside his office at a large, state-owned teaching hospital as he explained to her how he was going to remove a small, insignificant fibroadenoma (lump) from her breast the following day. He promised Sophie that her breast would be left intact for "there wasn't one chance in a million" that removal of the whole breast would be needed, as her tumor was benign.

The Professor was probably the best surgeon in Athens for diseases of the breast. Sophie had been told this, which filled her with a sense of security. She felt an even greater sense of reassurance because she had paid, in advance, an exorbitant fee specified by the Professor. The money, of course, was paid under the table.

In Greece, fees charged by physicians for health services are legitimate only in settings involving private-patients' cases in the private sector. Greece has "universal health care" subsidized by heavy taxation. Most physicians are salaried employees of the state, and as such are required to provide services to patients free of charge. If "black money" is requested under the table for any given procedure, it is considered a serious breach of state laws. What's more, if the request for payment is made prior to scheduling a procedure, and could result in a "black money" patient jumping ahead of other patients awaiting treatment, it is considered bribery or even blackmail by courts. Sophie felt that the large amount of money she had paid him secured for herself quality services of the highest standards possible.

Sophie had only been admitted two hours ago. All her preoperative laboratory tests were completed, thanks to the earnest efforts of a junior physician who was so instructed by the Professor. Thus, Sophie was prepared for the next day's "standard" procedure.

*She got up, shook hands with her surgeon and walked toward the door of his office. All of a sudden something on her brown case folder caught her eye. On the front of the folder, the Professor had just written her first name, surname, and the abbreviated phrase "**Ca** of breast." Instantly, Sophie felt as if she were engulfed in darkness as her vision faded. Thoroughly stunned by what she saw, she crumbled unconscious to the floor. She would have broken some bones upon collapsing if the junior physician hadn't held her.*

When she regained consciousness, she couldn't stop the tears brought on by memories of her beloved father. He had died of gastric cancer, and Sophie recalled that all his medical records displayed the very same "Ca" abbreviation as the main diagnosis. She understood that "Ca" meant "cancer." Sophie then remembered how everyone had lied to her father and had hidden his diagnosis from him, because that was considered the appropriate, decent way of doing things in the past. She only wished such hurtful, harmful old customs had been abandoned by now…after such a long time!

At once she lost all confidence in the Professor, as well as in her own husband. She no longer knew whom to trust or whose advice she should listen to. For a brief time, she wanted advice from no one at all. A grim thought took hold of her mind: she was alone, without any trustworthy allies while facing this monumental struggle, a fight that would call for brave decisions that must be based on true and accurate data.

How on Earth can physicians think that they alone understand the simple "coded" abbreviations of the English terms for Cancer (Ca) and Tumour (Tu)? Almost every citizen of this country has lost a relative, neighbor, or colleague during his lifetime to cancer; so, they've seen before and recognize and remember the ostensibly secret abbreviations "Ca" and "Tu" written on discharge summaries, sick leaves, early retirement pension documentation, etc. Is this a humane way for patients to become aware of their own cancer diagnosis, by suddenly recognizing the "hidden" meaning of simple abbreviations?

Sophie was strong and willing to do whatever it took to save her life. No liars, however, were allowed to stand by her. She demanded to be discharged from the hospital at once, and immediately initiated divorce proceedings against her husband. She chose to undergo mastectomy at another hospital, but no one ever discovered which one.

Continuation of Chapter 5

Information about every event or fact occurring in the universe (i.e., all information) is ineradicably recorded within the very fabric of space-time. Information cannot be destroyed, deleted, or sent to oblivion, but rather it is *eternal*, no matter how long hidden away. In the latter cases information remains coded in forms very hard to decipher, as was proven recently by recording gravitational waves from a cosmic event that took place over a billion years ago[*].

In other words, the truth, ultimately, is always revealed; it cannot possibly stay hidden forever. Finally, patients *will* come to know the secret of their own diagnoses either out of accidental disclosure (medical information unintentionally read or overheard by patients) or, possibly, because of symptoms of progression of their disease.

Families are very cautious and usually extremely careful about what is openly said during meals and other family gatherings or meetings to avoid accidental disclosure

---

[*] The actual collision of two black holes had occurred longer than one billion years ago, as was reported on 02/11/2016 by the LIGO (Laser Interferometer Gravitational–Wave Observatory) research team.

or unintentionally bringing a sensitive matter to light. For the same reason, families become overly secretive and frantically hide all insurance records or files, discharge summaries, recommendations for sick leaves, and medical certificates. They also limit to the extreme the number of persons who are made aware of "the secret" (the cancer diagnosis) to avoid leaking that knowledge to the patient. No matter how diligently and zealously the families strive to conceal, eventually some factor or parameter, both unforeseen and uncontrollable, will allow the truth to be revealed. It is so dictated by the immutable laws of physics, including entropy!

One cannot hide the onset of new symptoms (should the disease progress) from the affected patient. Also, impressive inscriptions on the façades of buildings or large signs at the entry of hospital departments are hard to hide: they bear revealing terms such as "Radiotherapy," "Oncology," "Chemotherapy," etc. When patients need the services of these specialized departments to treat their disease, they will inevitably see the signs and immediately understand the diagnosis is cancer. No matter how deep the patients had been kept in the dark, the truth will ultimately be revealed or deduced. Discovering the truth in such a way is infinitely more emotionally traumatic for the patient and less manageable than if he or she had been properly and appropriately informed from the very beginning.

Patients will justifiably get angered because they should have been informed of their condition as soon as the diagnosis was made. Thus, patients lose confidence in people...in members of their own families and / or physicians in general. The prospect of a patient experiencing inexpressible grief while simultaneously frustrated by his / her own family is inhumane and cruel. Such patients have no one to turn to for moral and emotional support, as the very people who could possibly offer badly needed support are no longer trusted. These patients experience the deep sorrow of being at once seriously ill and *feeling utterly alone*, which is much worse than merely suffering from cancer only. No family member can possibly desire to set his / her beloved relative in such a situation.

In the modern era, battles against cancer can often result in victory. Hope for cure truly exists. For papillary carcinoma of the thyroid gland, for example, the 5-year survival rate is a 93%, 10-year survival rate is 90%, and 20-year survival rate is 84%. Usually several "battles" are required to achieve a cure. Surgery and / or chemotherapy (with potentially toxic side effects) may be required. In other words, patients need to be courageous and determined;

they must possess the will to fight for life and be prepared to face whatever it takes to defeat their disease. The struggle will be demanding, for cancer is a tough adversary.

Since the fight against cancer is difficult enough as it is, there is hardly any justifiable reason for making things even harder by obscuring facts, hiding diagnoses, lying, or telling half-truths. Success in defeating cancer depends on the cooperation and concerted efforts of the patient, physicians, and relatives; one doesn't win wars alone or by deceiving one's allies or developing strategies based on inaccurate information.

Patients draw the strength to fight bravely from the support and comfort of their family and close friends. If patients are made aware of what they are about to face at the outset, they feel loved, respected, and appreciated, and a stubborn will grows within, encouraging them to fight for life with full faith and trust in their physicians as their helpmates. Well-informed patients understand from the beginning that treatment might include major surgery, and they're better prepared to accept it should surgery become necessary to save their lives. Knowing this up front avoids any cause for bitter feelings later on for having been deceived.

Casualties unfortunately do occur in all wars. But the patient-warrior is not alone in his fight when supported by trustworthy allies. Armed with the truth and prepared for the battle that lay ahead, the patient-warrior advances against the disease, lacking any fear of the unknown, and is cured!

6.

"Depression" Is One Thing. "Sorrow" Is Another.

Historic Fact

An aircraft crashed at noon on August 14, 2005 on a wooded area near "Grammatikon" village, in central Greece. It was the fatal HCY 522 flight, operated by Helios Airways from Larnaca, Cyprus to Athens, Greece. All on board perished, 121 souls in total, including 22 children. It would be a full day before a list of the deceased would be made public. The victims' families experienced long hours of emotional agony. They immediately rushed from Cyprus to Greece to look for their relatives, not knowing whether they were alive or dead.

Psychologists dashed to the scene to aid and "support" the newly arrived Cypriot relatives of flight HCY 522 passengers. These psychologists were dispatched by the legendary "Daphni Psychiatric

Hospital" in Athens according to a direct order by its Director. Yet the newly arrived Cypriots were neither mentally ill nor did they display any indication of "incongruous (or inappropriate) affect." They merely needed to know whether their loved ones were alive. They also wanted to be properly informed about the investigation of the tragedy by qualified officials of the authorities in charge. It may be also presumed they were seeking accountability and justice for the victims when all the facts involved in the tragedy were known.

It took nearly 10 years of lawsuits, trials, and appeals before the courts rendered final judgment: the crash of flight HCY 522 was a result of human error and negligence on the part of several defendants who were charged with manslaughter. All those convicted were punished by an ostensibly "custodial" sentence that was, however, commutable to approximately an € 80,000 fine; so, in effect, no real "custodial" sentences were served by physically doing time.

Bereaved mourners need human tenderness, compassion, and sympathy during times of great sorrow. The latter is an emotion that one normally and not unexpectedly feels whenever one experiences the loss of a dear loved one. "Sorrow" is not synonymous *with "depression," which is considered a disorder. An illusion is growing in modern society, wherein one who naturally grieves the loss of a loved one or suffers a catastrophic life event is diagnosed with depression. When natural human sorrow is misclassified as depression, psychiatrists and psychologists can justify need for treatment where none exists. The mental health community is "medicalizing" human feelings by turning normal emotions into "disorders."*

In our modern era, irresponsible people have been appointed to positions of great responsibility as officials at various agencies or institutions, or are placed in charge of them. Such officials do their very best to disclaim any responsibility or duty as human beings by attempting to avoid consoling those who mourn and expressing compassion, empathy, or sympathy. Instead, such duties are being transferred to mental-health professionals, who are to replace the proper officials of the controlling authorities, or so it seems that it is attempted. No spokesman or other representative of Helios Airways volunteered to face the victims' relatives to express condolences, to commiserate with them, to apologize for the tragedy, or shed tears. Neither did any other representatives, not even officials of the Civil Aviation Authority or experts of the committee investigating the tragedy.

Continuation of Chapter 6

During our lives, we all experience events that vary greatly in the degree to which they affect our emotions. We celebrate happy events; for instance, birthdays or personal successes in sports, at school, or professional accomplishments, etc. We're jubilant when we at last find our "better half," that special person who will bring happiness to our lives. We feel joy for our own children and take pride in their achievements. On the other hand, we experience deeply unpleasant emotions caused by events that are devastating to us; for instance, grief over the loss of loved ones, as well as material loss, loss of a job, or the catastrophic loss caused by destructive natural disasters caused by earthquakes, or major fires, for example.

It is normal, of course, to experience joy in response to the pleasant moments that brighten our lives; on the other hand, it is equally normal to feel sorrow in response to unpleasant events we all experience. It is imperative that we are able to unravel any confusion between sorrow and depression, which are two different things. Sorrow is an *emotion* normally experienced by any human being enduring a negative, unpleasant, or distressing event. We are entitled to feel sorrow when our mother dies, or when we discover that burglars have broken into our home, or when belongings are repossessed when payments are overdue.

Nowadays, however, the term " depression " is routinely abused so often it has become a cliché. It has come, inappropriately, to replace "sadness." "Depression" sounds more modern, and therefore attractive and "politically correct," to many people, including journalists, and pop-culture figures who gladly subscribe to cracker-barrel philosophy elaborated with an unbearable lightness*. The fact is that true depression is actually a *disorder*, dealt with by psychiatry and psychology. A patient suffering from true depression feels sad or negative emotions for no apparent reason at all.

For instance, a person earning a decent living, with a secure job, in no financial distress, who has suffered no serious loss of any sort—with everything in life really going smoothly—suffers from true depression, if he / she feels overly sad for no discernible reason. This person might feel sad to the point of being unable to function, but won't be

---

* The title of Milan Kundera's book "*The Unbearable Lightness of Being*" is herein quoted.

able to explain why. True depression is a psychologically abnormal condition that needs to be evaluated by an expert, such as a psychiatrist.

Likewise, there would also be an equally abnormal psychological condition present if one erupted in genuine laughter and celebrated when informed that he / she had cancer. The above-mentioned hypothetical situation is a severe symptom psychiatrists call "*incongruous* affect " (affective incongruity) or "*inappropriate* affect" ("inappropriate hilarity"). Obviously, if such a bizarre reaction occurs in response to deeply disturbing news, this patient definitely needs expert help.

On the contrary, it is inappropriate to diagnose someone with depression who feels sad after losing their job, or while going through an unwanted divorce, or after being diagnosed with cancer. In those cases, the person is merely responding reasonably to a serious stressor, and is reacting as one might expect a normal person would. Much can be done to help this person; the comfort of human compassion can be offered (the "milk of human kindness"), a hug might be welcomed, or a handkerchief to wipe away tears, to name a few common-sense gestures of sympathy. Ultimately, time will erase the pain, and the sufferer will re-emerge from the grip of sorrow.

Reemergence—or the *overcoming of sorrow*—means simply that one learns to cope with sorrow and moves on after *having first gone through it.* That is to say that one will inevitably have to first experience real, genuine sorrow in order to be able to overcome it. I go *through* sorrow to leave it behind me for good and to carry on with my course in life.

Patients who suffer from cancer will, yes, feel sad when informed of the diagnosis; there is nothing abnormal or unexpected about that initial emotional reaction. These patients will need their families', friends', or other helpmates' love, support, sympathy (even tears), understanding, and their encouraging words. They will finally need some time, too. Eventually, they will overcome sorrow by hopefully looking forward to the treatment, stepping foot on pathways of acceptance, or even merrier ones. It is rare that a total stranger—even an expert in psychiatry or psychology—can offer the balm needed for the cancer patients' sorrow if they lack a loving support system including friends and relatives.

Greek (and other countries') modern society has been indoctrinated to believe that everything is ostensibly doable, attainable, and feasible. Furthermore, the public believes it is easy to achieve everything without any effort, toil, fatigue, sweat, or worry. Such belief came from the evidently fraudulent—and obviously improbable—promises made by politicians. The latter promised the world to everyone: they pledged to hire all as employees, to have undersea tunnels dug, to remain in the Eurozone without sacrifices necessary to pay debts. The politicians even repeatedly pledged prosperity and well-being assured for all, by lying that "money does exist!" *. This society is also besotted after being brainwashed by marketing of goods and / or services to promote over-consumerism.

This society has long been trained to forget about realism and never to question the obviously absurd, unreasonable and impractical; it has been taught to accept anything as "possible," no matter how evidently fake or unrealistic it seems, on the condition that this accepted "anything" be pleasant. This society believes that the following miracle is feasible: that a patient may not feel sorrow at all—*not even for a brief instant*—when bad news breaks if it is a professional psychiatrist or psychologist

---

* Quotation from G. Papandreou Jr.'s speech during a TV debate prior to his winning the 2009 general election in Greece and becoming the first Prime Minister of the fiscal / financial crisis. Words that have managed to forever remain in Greek people's memory as an infamous synonym for politicians' lies.

who breaks it in some sort of magical way (bad news such as a cancer diagnosis or a relative's death or a divorce)!

Greek modern society is willing to pay considerable amounts of money as fees for professional experts' services as long as it is relieved from its dreary burden to break bad news. In our society, no one wants to become the bearer of bad news. "Cool" persons alone have a rightful place in the society, who fit under the "life and soul of the party" classification. It is unheard of or unfathomable for any member of this society to occasionally announce unpleasant facts; so, let someone else break the news, anyone else, even a hired professional!

During the author's professional life, patients' families often asked to call a psychiatrist merely to break the bad news. Yet human compassion alone was all that was finally necessary. No psychiatrist in the world can perform a miracle: it is impossible to undo or erase the causes of sorrow; no psychiatrist can resurrect a fellow passenger who died during the same traffic accident or make cancer disappear from a patient's body as by magic.

Of course, psychology claims to have identified *five stages* of mourning and grief: (1) Denial, (2) Aggression, (3) Bargaining, (4) Depression, and finally, (5) Acceptance!

One doesn't consciously choose to experience this series of emotions. The emotions are more or less subconscious defensive reactions that occur spontaneously as well as inevitably—at least some of them if not all and in any order—whenever one feels grief or sorrow caused by major loss (e.g., loss of employment, spouse, property, etc.).

Psychologists exist, of course, and their involvement, contributions, and support may well prove useful indeed; yet their involvement should never be considered either as substitute for human kindness and sympathy or as equivalent to the supportive compassion that only a beloved person can offer to a patient at a different level. Of course, psychiatric help is needed—even urgently—in cases of patients with "inappropriate or incongruous affect" as described earlier. Similarly, a psychiatrist's help is needed in cases of a pre-existing psychiatric disease or disorder.

At last, psychiatric involvement is needed for patients who express emotions of sorrow that are excessively intense as well as for patients who are locked in any of the above-mentioned five stages and cannot overcome it and move on.

The majority of patients can cope with sorrow and overcome it with emotional support from beloved friends and / or family under the responsible guidance and supportive advice of the attending clinician. The latter should have the necessary professionally acquired experience on how to effectively and appropriately offer supportive encouragement to patients who are understandably sorrowful, yet mentally healthy.

Patients above all else need the warmth of human emotional involvement, such as empathy and compassion, expressed by their physician as well as by their loved ones. Neither psychotherapy sessions nor antidepressant or sedative medications can substitute for, or replace, the human touch.

Religious patients can draw vast amounts of strength and hope from their faith. Such discussions, however, are beyond the scope of this book, which is written by a mere surgeon who treats human bodies, and who isn't a "healer of souls."

7.

Informed Consent

Clinical Counterexample

Peter had been a truck driver. During his retirement years he enjoyed drinking a little bit more than he did while employed, and he continued smoking as well. Before the Christmas holidays, he caught a cold and became hoarse. The hoarseness, however, persisted for far too long—more than 20 consecutive days since the onset of his cold symptoms. Peter's nephew, who was a year shy of receiving his medical degree, grew quite concerned; he insisted that Peter needed to be examined by a physician at the earliest possible date—before New Year's Day—and undergo laryngoscopy.

Laryngeal cancer was diagnosed without any spread or dissemination of the disease. Peter underwent surgery at a large teaching hospital in

Northern Greece. Peter's laryngectomy was successful. Of course, removal of the larynx, or "voice box," meant that Peter could no longer speak.

Prior to surgery, Peter's surgeon did not inform him that he had been definitively diagnosed with cancer or that he should expect to lose his voice. Hence, he postoperatively felt misled and betrayed.

Peter survived his cancer and lived another 20 years. But the loss of his voice caused profound emotional distress and he took to drowning his sorrow in drink. He couldn't possibly feel happy or even grateful—to God or for his good luck—about the favorable outcome achieved, because he ultimately rejected the initial diagnosis of cancer altogether. For fear of upsetting him, Peter's family did not inform him of the diagnosis until five years after his surgery.

He kept drinking on a daily basis, feeling sad, bitter, and cursing his nephew for talking him into undergoing examination and laryngoscopy. It was unfair to hold his nephew responsible for the ostensibly unnecessary loss of his speech. Peter should have been thanking him, of course, because it was indeed his nephew's prompt action that led to an early diagnosis and curative treatment! Strangely enough, Peter never expressed any complaints nor muttered any curses against the surgeon who had performed the procedure…without having first obtained his informed consent!

When Peter was eventually told the truth, many years later, he simply didn't believe it. He made that clear to his family in a blistering accusation written in his journal. His message read as follows: "You're lying to make up excuses for my cursed nephew, who wronged me. If I had really had cancer, I would have been dead by now. You either lie or the diagnosis was mistaken."

In Peter's mind a cancer diagnosis was ruled out by the fact that he was still alive. He always thought of cancer as a death sentence, and this perception persisted despite his own reality! He died some twenty years later of an unrelated cause, always complaining and without ever celebrating his victory or having felt any joy for his luck. Not even those in his social sphere ever knew that one of their own had been diagnosed with cancer, was cured of cancer, and survived 20 years in the small town in Thessaly, central Greece.

Peter was cured of cancer he didn't know he had thanks to a surgical resection that permanently deprived him of his speech.   He went into surgery, however, without being informed of, and consenting to, the known consequences of laryngectomy!

Continuation of Chapter 7

In every civilized country, the inviolability of human life is considered the premier legal good and must be protected at all costs. Citizens of liberal-legal civilizations enjoy freedom of contract, which means that any adult with "mental capacity" (being of sound mind) has the *inalienable* right to enter into a "legal deed" or "legal transaction" or "contract" with another party*. For instance, a sane adult (with "capacity") has the right to donate property (land or real estate as well as goods and chattels), the right to accept or to reject an offered donation, the right to redact a last will and testament, the right to contractually sell or to buy real estate property, etc.

In addition, every sane adult has the right to make crucial decisions—life and death decisions—regarding any subject that directly pertains to his or her body and life. Liberal-legal civilizations also recognize one's inalienable

---

* In Greek law, a "legal deed" is defined as the formal written expression of one's wish for the record in a valid and official way (usually witnessed and attested to by a notary or an attorney–at–law) that is legally binding. (In Greek: "δικαιοπραξία," pronounced "dhikeopraksia.")

right to give or refuse consent for medical and surgical procedures. After all, consent *is* merely another form of "legal deed."

It isn't customary even for a court of law to revoke one's "contractual rights" (rights to enter into legal deeds), even in a hypothetical case regarding the rights of a convicted criminal sentenced to capital punishment for particularly heinous acts (e.g., for serial murders, etc.). It is customary, however, for a Court to deprive one of certain civil rights (e.g., the right to vote). Hence, a convict retains the right to redact his / her last will and testament and to enter into legal deeds in general on the condition that he or she is a sane adult*.

Since "contractual rights" are not denied to criminals, it follows that no person is entitled to deprive another person of their rights to consent or refuse consent for treatments or procedures, as provided for by law. Therefore, if a patient's relative or relatives attempt to

---

* The requirements regarding "legal deeds" and one's rights to enter into them (one's "contractual rights") are covered by articles 128–130, 180, 1666 & 1668 of the Civil Code in Greece. More or less similar law principles are in force in most countries, usually with some variations in technical details.

intervene and act as the patient's agent—without that person's knowledge—and give their own consent and permission for major surgical resections, this is a blatant violation of principles of law even more grave than a merely unlawful act!

Hence, patients alone retain the exclusive right to express their own will for the record, formally and officially, and in a legally binding manner. It is the patients alone who have the right to grand consent (or to refuse), provided they are adults and mentally competent.

There is only one condition required by law for a patient's consent to be valid; the potential risks and benefits inherent in a given surgical procedure or any other medical treatment must have been clearly explained to the patient, and the patient must acknowledge that he or she understands the risks and potential benefits. Only under these conditions can a patient agree to and sign "informed consent."

In other words, a patient's consent for surgery is legally and actually *invalid* if the patient had been lied to about the true extent of the resection that is planned. For instance, a patient's consent is invalid for any planned "standard major resection of human organ" or similar surgical resection / amputation, if the consent was given on the understanding that only "a minor, limited, local debridement of a small abscess" was planned.

All surgical procedures are categorized as *"resectional"* if they remove (they "resect" or they take out) a normally present human organ (or a substantial part thereof). They are analogous to surgical amputation of an extremity, but their final result remains concealed instead*. Examples of resectional operations include the following: appendectomy, cholecystectomy (removal of the gall bladder), laryngectomy, hysterectomy (removal of the uterus or womb), pneumonectomy (removal of an entire lung), lobectomy (removal of a pulmonary lobe, the latter being a substantial part of a lung, usually measuring one third of the lung or half a lung), gastrectomy (removal of stomach), nephrectomy (removal of a kidney), splenectomy (removal of spleen), mastectomy (removal of breast), orchiectomy (removal of testicle), etc.

After surgical resection, some physiologic function is usually impaired or somehow impeded or hampered; loss of

---

* Any major surgical resection may be thought of as an "amputation" of an internal human organ, but the "amputation" term generally applies to an extremity (upper or lower) of the human body.

function can even be permanent. For instance, an "abdominoperineal resection" (a major surgical procedure for treating rectal cancer located in close proximity to the anus) removes the anus along with affected tissue of the rectum as a single surgical specimen. This procedure is associated with a significant chance of cure, but because the rectum and anus are removed, a new exit point for stool needs to be created in the lower abdomen. This new opening (called a stoma) is fitted with a colostomy bag that collects gas and stool. Thus, patients who undergo this procedure permanently lose the ability to pass stool via normal bowel movements*.

Similarly, laryngectomy results in permanent loss of natural speech (speech can be synthesized, however, using an artificial voice box or "Electrolarynx"), pneumonectomy results in some deterioration of respiratory function, total pancreatectomy causes diabetes and some digestive dysfunction as well (medications containing enzymes can be

---

* A cured patient will enjoy a long full life. A "colostomy bag" attached to the stoma at the front of his / her abdomen discretely collects the excreted solid refuse of digestion (feces). The bag is almost always concealed under clothing and doesn't interfere with usual social activities.

administered postoperatively to facilitate digestion), and so on.

No one wants to be deceived, to submit to general anesthesia under the false impression (or promise) of undergoing an ostensibly minor procedure of having a small fibroma removed from one's breast or lung, then wake to find out that the entire breast or lung has been removed. Yet even in our time there may be cases of relatives who consent to procedures, acting on their own as health-care agents, without the patient's knowledge or consent. If such deceitfulness is permitted to take place in our time, then it is an absolute disgrace for the medical and legal professions and every other aspect of our civilization!

The author is optimistic enough to hope that his colleagues worldwide take great care to ensure that *unambiguous informed consent* is properly obtained before performing any surgical procedure or administering any medical treatment associated with toxicity or any other serious risks. No patients are, however, expected to provide consent for major surgery if they were deceived by a falsified diagnosis: e.g., I won't give my consent as a patient to have my entire lung removed for ostensibly "debriding" a supposed "abscess" (or lesions caused by tuberculosis), since I know that a neighbor of mine was successfully cured from an abscess or tuberculosis with administration of antibiotics or other medication without surgery!

In the course of obtaining informed consent for treating cancer with surgery, patients are frequently asked to sacrifice an organ or a substantial portion of that organ in order to rid their bodies of their disease. Before asking patients to make such a sacrifice, they should have a thorough understanding of their confirmed diagnosis, the goal of treatment, and the risks and benefits involved so they are equipped to make a truly informed decision regarding consent. If patients are denied the truth, misled, or deceived in any way, any consents obtained would be meaningless, and a cycle of deceit would ensue in which physicians repeatedly and continuously try to justify lies with more lies, inevitably leading to inconsistencies until *they ultimately end up contradicting themselves.*

Of course, no reasonable person would consent to any major surgical resection or amputation if led to believe their disease is benign. If patients have no cause to think their condition is terribly serious, they will justifiably raise objections to major surgery. At that, the physician will endeavor to wear down their resistance, often helped by the patients' families (with the family being aware of the cancer diagnosis, of course). Thus, one lie leads to another as an excuse to force patients consent, until self-contradictory advice inevitably emerges, which the patients easily spot.

Clinical situations such as that mentioned above do not reflect well on any professional physician or other caregiver, if they occur, since they resemble attempts to pressure consumers to buy useless products by applying aggressive, heavy-handed marketing techniques!

It isn't only a matter of violation of the entirety of articles of penal law: average ordinary patients will eventually figure out they're being deceived. Unfortunately, this realization robs them of all confidence, leaves them feeling alone, wandering a confusing path without reliable guidance or the moral support of caregivers who can be trusted.

On the other hand, average ordinary patients who are aware of their true diagnosis, and therefore understand that their lives are at stake, are able to assess their situation accurately, weigh the pros and cons of whatever treatment or procedure is recommended by their physicians, and make an informed decision, no matter how difficult that decision may be. Well-informed patients, after weighing all the evidence and options, almost invariably choose life. They choose to proceed with the recommended treatment wholeheartedly, bravely, often bitterly, but they keenly fight without complaining much. They trust the honest, responsive, supportive people who fight alongside them.

Sane adult patients absolutely have *the right to refuse consent* to any treatment recommended provided they are aware of the potential consequences of their refusal. These consequences should be made crystal clear to the patients, explained frankly, and in full detail. This understanding is critical, for it is the patients themselves who will bear full responsibility for their decision.

In summary, hiding the true diagnosis *poisons* the entire therapeutic process, with justifiable objections raised by the patients, for *deception* is usually employed to convince or pressure them to submit to recommended treatment. If a series of punishable illegal acts occurred, it would lower medical professionals' level to the common criminals'. In such a case, patients would be deprived of their own inalienable and sacred human rights—the right to sovereignty over their own bodies and the right to have trustworthy supporters among their loved ones. No true humanitarian should ever wish that any of the above-mentioned scenarios should come to pass!

8.

Compliance and Follow-Up

Clinical Counterexample

You'll recall from the previous chapter's clinical counterexample the story of Peter, a man with laryngeal cancer who permanently lost his ability to speak after undergoing curative laryngectomy. He was not informed beforehand that this lifesaving procedure would cost him his voice. Nor, for that matter, was he informed that he was diagnosed with cancer. Consequently, Peter was extremely upset that this surgery was allowed to proceed without first obtaining his informed consent.

He should have returned for regularly scheduled follow-up examinations during the first five years after surgery so that potential disease recurrence might be detected early. Yet Peter, utterly unaware that he had cancer and that the disease could recur, declined any further examinations. Five years later his family finally told him he had cancer and that the surgery he underwent saved his life. Peter, however, didn't believe them; he was convinced they were either lying to him or that the initial diagnosis was incorrect.

In any case, during the remaining 20 years he survived, Peter would never again permit any medical practitioner to examine him. He wrote relentlessly in his journal, informing others of his loathing for physicians and reminding all that he didn't even want to be reminded of the existence of their self-serving, nefarious "cabal."

Continuation of Chapter 8

The previous chapter illustrated how difficult it can be to persuade a person in the general population to sign consent forms authorizing any potentially unpleasant treatment (e.g., resection or a therapy associated with toxicity) if the person is unaware that they have cancer. On the other hand, a person fully informed of their diagnosis might in fact be eager to undergo such treatment on the understanding that their very lives are at stake.

The uninformed patients' reasonable reluctance to provide consent is typically followed by a trail of problems, because each objection to treatment is usually met with a new ruse. The result is a cascade of lies devised to cover up inevitable contradictions caused by earlier lies offered in the relentless effort to obtain invalid "informed" consent. When the patients at last discover that they have been misled all along, they lose confidence in those once trusted.

In this chapter, we'll explore a further complication of withholding a cancer diagnosis from a patient. Let's suppose, hypothetically, that diagnosis-naïve patients were "somehow" convinced to provide consent for a given treatment. (For the purposes of this exercise, let's set aside for the moment all legal issues regarding the invalidity of a consent obtained based on lies, deception, and unawareness.) What happens after consent is granted under false pretenses?

Treatment that patients were persuaded—or even forced—to accept against their wishes will proceed. Surgical resection of an organ or amputation of an extremity will be carried out or chemoradiotherapy sessions will start. The patients will then experience various treatment–emergent adverse effects, which can be extraordinarily unpleasant (postoperative pain, draining catheters, nausea and vomiting, general malaise, etc.).

Subsequently, the patients will reasonably suspect that they're suffering needlessly. After all, they've been led to believe their disease was rather minor, mild, benign, or at the very least "nothing grave." They will see no reason for ordering treatments so unjustifiably potent and debilitating. As a result, they're likely to grow angry with those who had a hand in obtaining their consent.

These patients might *never again return*, of their own free will, to the hospital or institution for subsequent chemotherapy sessions. Such patients might refuse to comply with any physicians' orders whatsoever or even decline to continue taking medications. They won't understand that they really do need additional medication, or worse, think that it is the treatment itself that causes them to feel sick rather than their true (still unknown to them) disease.

Even in cases of patients not requiring postoperative adjuvant treatment, they will still need to be seen in regular follow-up for a specific length of time (generally five years). That is to say, patients will definitely need to keep up regular appointments to be re-examined according to a preset follow-up schedule (e.g., once every 3 or 6 months) until surveillance is completed and they are considered "cured."

The purpose of follow-up surveillance is to detect any possible recurrence of cancer early, before disease adversely affects the patient's quality of life. Early detection of recurrence may lead to additional therapeutic strategies or treatment options that could prove effective.

It only makes sense for a patient to reject further treatment or follow-up appointments if he believes he agreed to undergo surgery that was ultimately unjustifiable and sacrificed a limb or organ unnecessarily. Not only do such patients refuse further examination, but they also reject any further treatment, even if such postoperative (or "adjuvant") treatment is recommended to them.

Patients, who consider themselves deceived and exploited, of having been surgically robbed of their own flesh for incomprehensible reasons, will no longer feel any confidence; they don't comply with the recommendations of any physicians (even new ones) or trust the advice of their own relatives. They consider the latter guilty of manipulating them to sign a forced consent; it was their relatives, after all, who helped persuade the patients to deviate from their initial objections.

Thus, withholding a cancer diagnosis not only poisons the whole therapeutic effort during its delivery, it may cause early discontinuation of chemotherapy sessions or noncompliance with other medical advice or follow-up schedules. Those who supposedly endeavor to "avoid causing sadness" to patients by deceiving and withholding a diagnosis inevitably do so at the expense of the very person they hope to help.

9.

Half-truths, Evasion and Jargon

Clinical Counterexample

Clio was struggling to recall the precise words her physician used when he informed her of her diagnosis. It sounded as though he said something like "measly epithelioma." Or was it "measles epithelioma"? The latter couldn't be correct; she saw no evidence of skin rash nor was she feverish. It really didn't matter, Clio happily thought, because she didn't hear "cancer" or "carcinoma" mentioned in any context when he gave her the news. Thus, she was malignancy-free.

Or so she thought.

Clio was a middle-aged, uneducated farmer who sought medical advice after developing a chronic pain that spread across the ribs of one side of her chest. The ache grew nastier at the slightest cough, sneeze, or when taking a deep breath. In addition, she often became short of breath with relatively minor exertion. Her doctor called the last symptom "dyspnea." He discovered fluid had accumulated in her chest cavity and drained it with a pleural tap using a needle. Softly she spoke, within earshot of her doctor, "thank God, my biopsy only showed this 'measly' thing…with the strange name, and there's nothing serious going on."

The proper medical term for her diagnosis was, unfortunately, "mesothelioma." It was a term Clio never heard before; she was utterly unaware that it described a type of malignant neoplasm, quite difficult to treat, with an ominous prognosis. Her doctor neither explained what the term meant nor discussed the gravity of her situation. Quite the contrary, in fact, he was cheerful and smiling when he mentioned her diagnosis, as if the latter were too insignificant for her to be worried about!

Yet Clio's children and husband started exhibiting unusual behavior after her health problem was diagnosed. They no longer allowed her to take part in day-to-day work in the fields. Even stranger, her family began stripping the asbestos shingles from their barn, which was also used for storage. Moreover, they themselves all made appointments to undergo chest x–rays and have other tests performed.

Clio didn't know what was going on, but she knew she didn't like it. Something wasn't right; something didn't make sense or fit. And Clio wasn't so easily fooled; she suspected she would soon learn more about this disease of hers with the strange name because her doctor's cheerful demeanor seemed over the top to her…out of place. Especially when recalling the tears she had glimpsed on her husband's face.

Continuation of Chapter 9

Numerous detailed arguments have appeared in this book against the deleterious practice of withholding the true diagnosis of cancer from patients. Counterexamples have also been provided to demonstrate how catastrophic the consequences of shielding patients from the truth can be. I have consistently emphasized that the appropriate course of action is to tell patients the truth while offering much-needed support and hope at the same time. All of the above aren't enough, though. In this chapter I will argue how important it is to explain diagnoses to patients using terms and language they will be able to *understand*.

It isn't acceptable for any doctor to cavalierly tell patients that a "tiny bit of cancer" is present inside their body, and using jokes or word play to diminish the perceived severity of their condition. In these early years of the 21st century, cancer still remains a serious disease. To ensure the best possible outcomes in treating malignancy, one must take the matter seriously and focus maximum attention on achieving cure, or at least maximizing the chances for it. In most countries, average adult patients are well aware of that fact.

So, if patients sense their own doctor trying to sound too casual, playful, or matter-of-fact about such a dreadful diagnosis, then they really start wondering whether they're dealing with a physician who might be irresponsible, imprudent, or merely foolish. The patients neither rest assured nor relaxed after such a glib manner of disclosure. They don't feel that they can rely on a physician who would behave so.

Why on earth would any responsible physician attempt to downplay the seriousness of such a diagnosis while initially breaking bad news to a given patient? Inexperienced or ignorant colleagues may attempt to blend parts of the truth along with lies so that their final verdict— soon to be revealed—might sound less painful than it really is as they attempt to provide encouragement and support to the patient. Most colleagues' intentions are benevolent; they truly do not intend to upset their patients or leave them despondent.

Some colleagues harbor ambitions to climb higher up the ladders of professional organizations or societies; they're eager to be elected to Councils or to chair Medical Associations etc. Moreover, some even aspire to positions of raw political power outside the medical community. Indeed, many of my colleagues have been elected to serve as mayors, Members of Parliament, Congressmen, or Cabinet Members in many countries. Politicians (including former practicing physicians) are notorious for possessing an innate tendency to avoid acknowledging any bad news or inconvenient, unpleasant truths. This common adaptive strategy among politicians is designed to avoid displeasing their constituents. They strive hard always to be pleasant to all, downplay the negative, and accentuate the positive. To achieve this they require verbal camouflage; they coin grandiose expressions for "sensitive" ears, consisting largely of euphemism in order to take the curse off blunt, perfectly acceptable terms. Thus, "garbage collectors" become "waste disposal engineers," the "town dump" is now the "volume reduction unit," and "cancer" withers into a "wee structural alteration."

Yet the modern era is defined by easy access to almost every kind of information imaginable, easily retrieved by powerful, increasingly sophisticated search engines on the Internet, such as Google, and founts of knowledge like Wikipedia and similar digital encyclopedias. The patients can, will, and do seek information about the nature of their diagnosis, which was downplayed during the initial disclosure by their physician*. And, usually, they will discover the truth in its entirety. This will cause a seismic shift in terms of confidence and, as well, threatens compliance with therapeutic advice.

Hence, any evasions, equivocations, subterfuge, or worse yet, making light of or joking about a serious diagnosis, offers neither support nor comfort to patients. On the contrary, such strategies repel the patients by making them more suspicious, guarded, reserved, and reticent. Any attempts to distract them from their concerns by adopting an insouciant attitude and overly relaxed body language may well trigger similar wariness. People are able to sense pretense, and when they detect suspicious signs and signals, they instinctively, if perhaps subconsciously, worry about being misled.

---

* In addition, so much information available on the Internet is in fact disinformation, or bad, misleading material. One can't expect all patients to be able to discern quality information from quackery. It isn't hard to find websites offering special information about cures "your doctor doesn't want you to know about!" This sort of claim might seem especially convincing to a patient who knows for certain that his doctor did indeed possess information he didn't want him to know about, and deliberately withheld.

Sometimes, physicians try to mask the severity of a diagnosis by using terminology unfamiliar to the nonprofessional. Many malignant diseases bear names that lack the familiar endings "-carcinoma" or "cancer." For instance, mesothelioma, osteosarcoma, seminoma, retinoblastoma, lymphoma are malignant diseases. Doctors who stick to formal medical terms, while technically correct, may hope they're able to hide behind a word unknown to their patient, much like the professor who abbreviated "Ca" instead of writing "cancer" on the front of Sophie's folder (in Chapter 5, pp.37–40) because he thought his Greek patient didn't speak English.

Resorting to half-truths about the recommended treatment (and its adverse effects) will have equally disastrous consequences. Patients may indeed be deceived enough to sign a consent form for a major surgical resection while under the impression it's a "routine, standard procedure." Patients may be completely unaware of the life-altering effects of abdominoperineal resection on the passing of stool via "normal" bowel movements, or the effects of pancreas resection on digestion and regulation of blood sugar levels, and so on. If a patient agrees to a procedure not having been fully informed of the risks and any known treatment-related adverse effects, then the consent form signed will be totally invalid, worth less than the cost of the paper it was printed on. The document will have been signed under false pretenses.

Let's say a few things about all "routine, standard procedures." Some conniving colleagues may describe major resectional surgery as ostensibly "routine" or "standard" when attempting to persuade patients to grant written consent. If such tactics are used, it is a clear case of unethical verbal slight of hand, since each and every procedure ever performed on any human being must by definition be considered "standard."

A surgical procedure is defined as "standard" if it has been accurately described in humans as a step-by-step sequence, in great technical detail, and with known benefits far outnumbering the risks, whenever performed for specific indications. Further, the technical detailed description of the "routine, standard" procedure must have been published in a recognized text book or reference book, unanimously approved as established by all clinicians in a field (vs. anecdotal case reports appearing as bibliography / refer-ence notes after experimental research). The risks of any routine, standard procedure must be absolutely known or reported as well as their possibility of occurring. Finally, the indications for carrying out the procedure must also be absolutely clear and unanimously accepted. So too must any possible contraindications to the procedure. Any deviations are strictly prohibited by medical ethics as well as by law in all modern, well-governed democratic countries.

Furthermore, experimenting or testing on humans is strictly prohibited in modern society. The use of animal models is allowed instead, but only under conditions strictly controlled in the setting of experimental operating theatres properly supervised by competent authorities. That is to say that no surgical procedure is allowed to be experimentally tested on human beings. In other words, each and every surgical procedure approved for humans must fall under the definition of "standard." This includes any procedure that some "clever" colleague might endeavor to gain consent for by describing it as "standard" or "routine." It is implied that all surgical procedures, from appendectomies to heart transplants, are conducted using "standard" procedures. Hence, describing a procedure as "standard" or "routine" is, in fact, *redundant* and can be *misleading*. The ill-advised patient who is told only that his procedure is considered "standard" can easily be lulled into an unwarranted level of complacency.

The truth is there's no such thing as an "absolutely risk-free" procedure—major or minor, surgical or medical. Even the oral administration of a pill or capsule of antibiotics might cause death due to allergic reaction or anaphylactic shock; a tonsillectomy may result in aspiration of blood due to uncontrolled bleeding.

Of course, major procedures are expected to be associated with even graver risks; patients with cancer are willing to accept these risks and provide consent to such procedures, often without reservation, because the stakes are high: they're engaged in a life-or-death struggle with the assistance of trusted allies. The allies are defined as such if honesty is their best and only policy.

I illustrate and explain the meaning of any and all esoteric medical terms to my cancer patients by using plain words as often as possible. For even greater clarity, I offer examples. The examples must draw from the given patient's professional or social experience—imagery he can relate to in his own life. I clearly and directly explain the nature of the disease without resorting to any diagnostic jargon that a patient may not know or comprehend, and the news is delivered with appropriate measures of solemnity, frankness, empathy and compassion.

I enumerate the specific risks known to be associated with the treatment indicated in the patients' case. In seeking informed consent, I offer compelling arguments in favor of treatment when I believe the potential benefits outweigh the potential risks and consequences of the necessary sacrifice (of an organ, usually, or an extremity) in order to save their life. I ease their anxiety and fear (of nondisclosure or deceit) and I disabuse them of their mistaken excessive fears. We move forward together, patient and physician; we strive to achieve cure, a goal demanding focus, consistency, and reassuring professional bearing.

Cancer patients don't like being trifled with, playing with half-truths, or being conned; they can spot inappropriate levity, redundant deceptions, and verbal camouflage. They want to fight for their lives and win with the help and support of trusted team mates. Along with kindness, they deserve the truth, our empathy, highest respect, and even awe. Finally, adults deserve to be treated as adults, not immature children who might be distracted from life's misfortunes by using antics designed to amuse or distract a frightened child.

10.

Who Should Disclose The Diagnosis

Clinical Counterexample

The reader may remember Magdalene's story in Chapter 2. She was admitted to a large teaching hospital on the day before undergoing major surgery (abdominoperineal resection) for colon cancer. Magdalene had been told absolutely nothing at all about her true diagnosis by her family to avoid causing her any more sadness (she had recently become a widow and was very much concerned about who would take care of her young daughter, who suffered from a rare autoimmune disease, if anything happened to her).

Prof. Argyris Papantoniou, her attending surgeon, hadn't informed her that she had cancer or about the major, unavoidable change to her body that would occur after the procedure; for the rest of her postoperative life Magdalene would have a surgically created opening in her abdomen (called a "stoma") through which stool would pass as opposed to natural presurgical bowel movements. A discrete "colostomy bag" would always be connected to the stoma that would remain concealed under her clothing. It was necessary to surgically remove the anus, too, as that tissue was also cancerous. The professor was to perform a major resection on his patient the following day, yet he hadn't informed her about the certain postoperative loss of her ability to defecate naturally.

Magdalene was twice blessed. A distant relative of hers passed by to wish her "good luck with the surgery" the evening before the operation; he happened to be a doctor himself, albeit of an altogether different specialty. He spent a couple of hours with her, during which time he gently informed her about everything her surgery entailed and what she should expect afterward. Moreover, he successfully persuaded her to change her mind after she initially rejected the idea of living with a stoma.

Finally, Magdalene was also lucky because she was cured of cancer, thanks to the successful resection undertaken by Prof. Papantoniou. She remains alive, *well, and disease-free as these words are being written, some 19 years after her surgery. In 2002, she was formally declared "cured." She always felt happy and grateful for being cured, and she considered the resection of her anus worth the sacrifice. Fortunately, Magdalene had the chance to consent to the procedure fully informed of what was being done and what to expect postoperatively. Consent was not extracted in her case from a position of ignorance.*

Continuation of Chapter 10

I have thus far attempted to expose the host of overwhelming problems caused by hiding or suppressing the true diagnosis from the patient. In the previous pages plenty of clinical counterexamples made clear the absurdity of conspiring to withhold a diagnosis from the very patient involved: problems of obtaining legitimate informed consent (as a result of willful deception), harms related to the patient's noncompliance with therapeutic advice or with regular follow-up schedules, erosion of confidence and reliance (both lost when the truth eventually or incidentally comes to light), and major issues concerning safeguarding the patient's interests from potential exploitation at the hands of cunning individuals known to the person, perhaps even family members, who might harbor selfish ulterior motives.

I have also attempted to explain by way of counterexamples and arguments why some ways of disclosing the diagnosis are harmful, especially if they are based on half-truths or evasions or are concealed behind incomprehensible terminology.

Finally, arguments have been presented showing that it is not necessary to involve psychiatrists or psychologists when informing patients about their diagnosis. Of course, there is a caveat to this—it is far better for patients to be made aware of their diagnosis, even if disclosed by a psychiatrist, than to be left utterly unaware about their condition.

In the next chapters an appropriate approach will be proposed regarding how best to break bad news to the patient. In this chapter, however, I will address the question of Who ought to be the one to break bad news. Who should disclose the diagnosis is a matter of paramount importance!

It is obviously the patient's own *attending physician* who should inform the patient; in fact, the physician is required by law to do so, as well as by medical ethics. Doctors have an absolute obligation to disclose the diagnosis to the very patient who had trusted them. The unbreakable bond between physician and patient can be based on nothing less than mutual honesty. Furthermore, physicians must have received training and clinical experience in how to appropriately and professionally disclose unpleasant diagnoses.

It is unseemly for doctors to accept only reward—fees, praise, fame, recognition—for anything good (easy-to-treat cases or when pleasant outcomes are expected), but to disclaim responsibility and avoid accountability when bad things happen (hard-to-treat or unpleasant cases). Elementary knowledge of ancient standards of medical ethics warrants consistency; the attending physician either "attends" all aspects of patients' care, both easy and hard, or he / she is not "attending" at all. These tenets also warrant principled conduct; attending physicians should be there, present, standing beside their patients always, for better (easy cases with pleasant outcomes) or worse (difficult cases with unpleasant information to announce)! The above-mentioned obligations arise from the very calling and function of medicine; they're the embodiment and quintessence of this profession.

It's hardly advisable for family members or other close relatives to disclose the diagnosis, since they haven't received training on how to do so and because they usually lack any practical experience. They simply don't know the appropriate way and, therefore, resort to impromptu attempts to extemporize. It is not right, though, to disclose serious information of paramount importance in an amateurish, slipshod, or haphazard way to patients; they will soon need to weigh the information very carefully while considering important decisions!

In cases where bad news is broken by close relatives, they may feel so stressed that they attempt to blend partial truths with lies to soften the blow. Partial lies, however, can later foster distrust and irreparable loss of confidence in other family members or caregivers; lies can also lead to problems with loneliness, as earlier explained.

It is worth noting that, in the first place, no relative should become aware of a cancer (or any other) diagnosis without the involved patient's prior permission. Patients alone can relieve their attending clinician from the confidentiality obligations relating to their diagnosis. Per medical ethics, the patients involved should be made aware of the diagnosis first; it is only after the patients grant unambiguous and explicitly expressed permission that their physicians can disclose a diagnosis to any other person, no matter how closely related. There's one only condition for the validity of the last sentence: the patients must be adult and legally sane.

One can, therefore, consider that attending physicians are guilty of ethical lapses if they perpetually defer informing their patients; physicians may be considered even more guilty if they fail to disclose the diagnosis altogether, in violation of their ethical obligation. Of course, no one expects doctors to be enthusiastic about breaking bad news. It is, however, their professional duty to do so and in an appropriate, humane manner!

Patients' families might turn to the thoughts of the last two paragraphs to exert pressure on reluctant attending physicians; this way the attending physician may well be persuaded to duly fulfill his / her obligation of informing the patient in a proper, appropriate, and professional way!

Patients' families may consider exerting such pressure as being justified, or even demanded, as a last resort to protect their loved ones from messy disclosures by unqualified third parties. After all, the pressure will only be exerted for purposes of prompting necessary action to be taken precisely as stipulated by the Laws of "The Art," the term Hippocrates used for "medicine."

The author concedes—as a necessary evil or compromise—that patients are better off being informed of the diagnosis even by their own family members (no matter how inexperienced or unknowledgeable they may be) rather than to remain in the darkness of wholesale ignorance.

At least their families do genuinely care about them and hold them in true feelings of loving kindness and affection.

11.

How to Break Bad News: 1ˢᵗ Session

The time has come to elaborate on the appropriate way to inform a patient of an unpleasant diagnosis. It is important to emphasize that the diagnosis should only be disclosed *when* it has been confirmed cytologically or by other definitive means, to the extent that *no clinical doubt* exists as to its accuracy. In prostate cancer, for example, secondary metastases found on bone scintigraphy can be diagnostic of a large, yet-to-be histologically documented, primary tumor.

According to Baruch Spinoza and other philosophers, an infinite series of ideas constitute "infinite intellect" (or "God's mind," as Spinoza otherwise defined it). In other words, infinite pathways to obtaining knowledge must exist, since knowledge itself is infinite. This leads me to believe that infinite pathways are available for physicians to follow as they lead their patients to knowledge of their diagnosis.

To reach the final destination point "A" (patient Awareness) from starting-point "I" (patient Ignorance), physicians may need to navigate several different pathways, passing through intermediate points (B, C, D, etc.) along the way. A clear, straightforward route may be the correct choice for a given physician, depending on his or her style or personality, when dealing with a receptive patient. More elaborate paths may be necessary, however, when dissimilarities between a physician and patient (in personality, temperament, etc.) make effective communication more challenging.

Every physician formally acquires the necessary condensed knowledge of how to break bad news to patients over the course of many years of undergraduate medical studies (no fewer than 6 years in Greece), throughout postgraduate training, and at least an additional 6–7 years of specialty training. Moreover, physicians attend continuing medical education seminars that often feature lectures with titles like "How to Break Bad News to Patients," as I did during specialist-training in the United Kingdom.

Beyond theoretical knowledge gained of how to inform patients, physicians also acquire priceless clinical experience during years of practice. Every physician develops a unique, highly personal style or "voice" that they use when delivering bad news to their patients, especially when that news involves cancer.

I would not, under any circumstances, claim special knowledge of how best to break bad news to patients. Myriad effective approaches, manners, and styles are practiced, the number of which may well approach the number of recognized "schools of thought" and accepted tenets of the Art of Medicine. Or it may, in fact, be fair to propose that the number likely equals the number of practicing physicians in the world! My own personal approach of informing patients will be described below; it has proved useful throughout my 33 years of clinical experience, and it continues to evolve as I constantly seek to improve upon what I've learned over those years.

Four sessions are usually necessary for informing a patient about an unpleasant diagnosis. An absolute minimum of twelve hours (at least) must pass between sessions. An even longer interval is highly desirable and recommended, because it allows patients time to reflect on and absorb the news of their diagnosis, as well as to vent intense emotions that invariably accompany the shock of learning one has cancer. Moreover, longer intervals also allow subconscious defense mechanisms much-needed time to run their course and at last allow the patient to accept the diagnosis. Unfortunately, allowing lengthy intervals between sessions is not always clinically feasible in some serious cases, especially if therapeutic or staging procedures are promptly required.

In rare instances of even greater clinical urgency (e.g., if a rescue or salvage procedure is necessary), two consecutive sessions can be combined. For instance, when clinical urgency is an overriding factor, a disclosing physician can offer sessions 2 and 3 as a single session. Caution is advised regarding the last session, however, as medical ethics forbids combining the 4th session with the previous (3rd) session!

The 1st Session is *preparatory*. The objective is to break the news gently, taking care to avoid overwhelming an unsuspecting patient who is wholly unprepared psychologically to handle the shock.

During this session, therefore, attending physicians should employ appropriate "body language," using gestures and postures consistent with an extremely concerned, serious person. There is no room at a moment like this for glib remarks, jokes, or a lighthearted attitude. The physician is obligated to wear the reassuring *mien* of a serious, thoughtful professional.

During the 1ˢᵗ Session the attending physician should never talk about cancer directly, but instead use *nonverbal cues* suggesting that they're engrossed in, or slightly distracted by, deep thoughts of their own regarding the case as they interact with the patient. The disclosing physician might use language like this:

> *We've discovered a "shadow" in your left lung that, frankly, has us concerned. All possible diagnoses—both better and worse—are under consideration right now. Until we know more, we can't rule out any of them.*

The physician should refrain from mentioning 'cancer' (or any of its derivatives or synonyms), not even by negative reference (i.e., denying it). In the unlikely event that the patient specifically asks whether cancer is possible or suspected during the 1ˢᵗ Session, the appropriate response might sound like this:

> *Please! I never said that. However, since you ask, I have to be honest with you. The truth is we can't rule out that possibility…for the time being at least. I know you're anxious right now, but please try to be patient while we wait for the pathology results to come back; then, we'll know exactly what it is we're dealing*

with. And I want to assure you right now, we have highly effective treatments today...for whatever the final diagnosis turns out to be. I'm confident of that. You're in good hands, and we'll be there for you, and with you, every step of the way.

Ample hope, in generous doses, must always be provided during all sessions and in every stage of disclosing the diagnosis. No disturbing words, especially "cancer," should be spoken during the 1st Session that might trigger fear or panic in the unprepared patient. Facial expressions and body language alone are used to "whisper" gently to the patient's soul and subconsciously prepare him / her to receive the news.

12.

How to Break Bad News: 2nd and 3rd Sessions

2nd Session

The 2nd Session advances patients *deeper* into the process of subconsciously *preparing* them psychologically to accept the reality of their diagnosis.

During this session, of course, attending clinicians should continue to comport themselves with the same air of concerned professionalism as described in the previous chapter; i.e., they should continue using the same body language, using gestures and postures consistent with the disposition of a profoundly concerned, serious-minded physician. Facial expressions and nonverbal gestures, again, should reveal a person who is deeply concerned, pensive, and sincere. During the 2nd Session, the physician further expands on the discussion initiated in the 1st by using *more direct* language. In other words, the physician begins to refer to the word "cancer," if only in an oblique, incidental context for the time being.

Of course, the physician is in an extremely delicate position, since the gradually increased level of candor required in session 2 is bound to provoke a degree of heightened apprehension in the patient. The doctor's facial expressions and body language, *must* project the persona of a confident clinician addressing an unfortunate situation. During these sessions, he must set aside and block any cheerful thoughts and emotions that might be associated with events in his personal life at the time. On the inside, for example, he might be celebrating the birth of a new grandchild; but such joy must not be allowed to surface during disclosure sessions. The obvious need for the physician to maintain an atmosphere of empathetic solemnity during such emotionally charged moments is essential to enabling the patient's subconscious defense mechanisms.

Some physicians may agonize over the thought of having to break news that's sure to cause their patients to worry. Nevertheless, it's an unavoidable responsibility—they must do so from time to time. While it's wonderfully satisfying when a physician can announce good news to patients, bad news is inevitable. And when it strikes, the physician must be there physically and emotionally for the patient, especially when severe, potentially catastrophic illness is diagnosed.

One needs to emphasize that no acting ability is required while disclosing a diagnosis. The facial expressions of profound concern for the patient come naturally, as do the physician's nonverbal gestures and mannerisms. Combined, they reveal the demeanor of a sympathetic, understanding professional, fully engaged with a patient enduring an intensely distressing moment. No theatrics are needed. The physician's heart is truly troubled by the knowledge that must be disclosed, and he or she feels genuine compassion for their patient.

One doesn't yet fully proceed to verbal and direct disclosure of the diagnosis in its entirety during this session, no matter how insistent the patient might be. One might address such a patient as follows:

Results of the CT scans and other tests are all back, and I'm afraid there's cause for more concern today regarding the nature of the mass in your lung than there was yesterday. I explained to you that various diagnoses, including cancer among other things, are currently being considered. We still can't rule out any diagnosis, for the time being at least. Not to worry too much, though: an altogether different diagnosis may eventually come to light. In any case, please remember this: we'll treat your disease, and we'll fight hard, no matter what it turns out to be, as there are plenty of effective treatments available today, for just about everything.

A patient does know about his / her own diagnosis—on a deeper, subconscious level at least—immediately after the 2nd session; there can be no doubt about that. Hence, all defensive mechanisms go into action, and they guide the patient through the "five stages of mourning and grief," as described in chapter 6 (on p. 56). At least some of these stages—if not all of them—are inevitable; the earlier they begin the process, the sooner the patient may come to "Acceptance" of the diagnosis.

A full day should be provided to the patient after the 2nd Session, if clinically feasible, to permit optimal psychological preparedness. During this stage, the patient is likely to weep, to show signs of worry, and, finally, to need emotional and moral support from family and friends as well as from nursing and allied support staff if he / she happens to be an in-patient at the time of disclosure.

It is best if a patient happens to be an in–patient when the diagnosis is revealed, as he / she has the benefit of remaining in a controlled, supportive environment under supervision of competent hospital staff during initial stages of adjustment. The patient is likely to have overcome initial distress by the time he or she is discharged. If so, the patient can resume normal social activities in an improved psychological state versus being sent home reeling from shock immediately after receiving devastating news.

3rd Session

The 3rd Session involves *full frank disclosure* of the diagnosis of cancer (or any similarly unpleasant disease). Of course, each doctor's personal style or voice will dictate how he / she directly and briefly will inform the patient. The doctor will speak calmly, in a serious voice, with respect, and as casually as possible. Candor is very important during the disclosure to save patients from prolonged anguish.

The doctor stands as the patient enters the office, shakes hands and gently touches the patient's shoulder for an instant. A comfortable seat or chair is offered to the patient. Without undue delay, the physician proceeds to break the news using only as many words as necessary, perhaps like this:

Jim, I've got the biopsy report back, and I'm afraid it shows some cancer cells inside the mass in your lung. So, we are dealing with cancer. Don't worry though, because there's some good news, too [in an emphatic voice]: this type of cancer responds Well to treatment. Hence, there is effective treatment we can offer you, Jim, and we expect your disease to

*respond to therapy. There's much we can do, and with
your consent, we'll fight this tumor with you side by side.*

Of course, "cancer" is mentioned without emphasis, but it is nevertheless repeated as often as necessary so the patient can become accustomed to hearing it.

Along with bad news, physicians are obligated to offer *hope* as well. We must discuss *curative* treatment, but only *if* the patient is a candidate for such treatment and realistic cause for hope exists for achieving a cure for this particular patient's disease stage and tumor type.

Even in cases where the prognosis is not as favorable as desired, we must still offer realistic hope. Then the vaguer term "treatment" should be used alone, instead of "curative treatment." It isn't dishonest when a physician promises they can "treat" the patient's cancer, unless they knowingly promise something they can't deliver; i.e., curative intent that isn't feasible. The physician is free to discuss and propose only those therapies indicated for a given patient's case, based on patient characteristics, performance status, disease stage, comorbidities, etc. In the majority of such cases (up to 99%), treatment involves either administering chemotherapy or employing multimodality treatments (e.g., surgery and adjuvant chemotherapy or radiotherapy).

Physicians are obligated to offer optimism and comfort to patients even in cases involving an unfavorable (or even a hopeless) prognosis, but they have no right to lie, at least not blatantly or in essence. In real life, to offer hope and comfort without lying is easier said than done. Physicians may make sincere promises to patients if they use flexible terms such as "therapeutic support" or "we can and will *help* you" versus the potentially misunderstood, more promising term "treatment." Once again, this isn't lying; palliative therapies—effecting adequate pain relief, prolonging life, and improving quality of life—constitute genuine humanitarian medical care.

At the risk of boring the reader, I must reemphasize: We do *not* lie to patients, because lies can and will cause them greater harm in the long run than any transient "relief" or the cruelty of false hope wrought by lies ever will.

One cannot emphasize enough that medical ethics *forbid* physicians to request consent for any form of treatment during the 3rd Session. It is expected that patients will be shocked by the news and emotionally stressed to the point that they aren't capable of comprehending fully the reality of their situation. Their minds will block their ears, allowing no unpleasant news to reach them.

A physician will be lucky if he manages to get a single piece of information to reach a patient's soul; this essential bit of knowledge is that *hope does* exist—whether a vaguely defined treatment in general or a curative treatment, which can and will be provided. For the time being, it is the most critical piece of information that one could sow inside of the patients' soul.

One doesn't elaborate *at all* on technicalities (various given ways of treatment or of their relative benefit–to–risk ratio) immediately after the disclosure of the diagnosis. No patient can be expected to have remained composed enough to be able to calmly evaluate options and to weigh significant parameters against one another at this stage. One has no right at this stage to expect patients to make their minds up and, finally, to reach critical, life-and-death decisions about a particular approach for treating their cancer (either surgically or non–surgically).

Immediately after disclosure, patients are expected to feel profoundly distressed emotionally; they frequently shed tears. They need clear signs of their doctor's compassion and empathy: a soothing word and supportive encouraging words, a handkerchief to wipe away tears, a glass of water, a brief touch on their shoulder!

The patients need even greater moral support from family, friends, and nursing staff! Loved ones are to be present with patients for many hours after disclosure, rather than leaving them alone immediately or shortly thereafter.

Family members who possess no medical knowledge (i.e., who don't know any better) are permitted to tell minor, trivial falsehoods, or "little white lies" while trying to encourage and comfort the patient, if their conscience permits. Yet no flagrant, blatant or unrealistic lies are encouraged, for these can cause catastrophic consequences in the future!

Combination of Sessions When Necessitated by Urgency

A full day's time at least *must* be allowed to elapse after the 3rd Session in all cases prior to the last, 4th Session. During that 4th Session the patient will have to choose between the various treatment options, after receiving and understanding detailed information about the pros and cons associated with each of them. It is highly desirable and recommended to allow even longer than one day's interval between the 3rd and 4th Sessions if possible; sometimes, however, this isn't practical or feasible.

In rare cases, there is no time to spare, because of an urgent need for decision-making. For instance, if the patient's life (i.e., the "premier legal good") is in immediate danger. In such rare cases, the disclosing doctor may need to combine two consecutive sessions (with a supposed interval between them) into one session. It is usually the 2nd Session that can sometimes be combined with the 3rd; in fewer cases the 1st Session can be combined with the 2nd.

Only once in my professional life did I have to speed up disclosure so that Sessions 1–3 had to take place in one day: This was a rare, desperate case where the utmost clinical urgency was needed. The first two sessions were combined as one session alone during the morning; the 3rd Session took place later in the afternoon of the very same day. Every aspect of news breaking was rendered even harder, uncomfortable, and more distressing for all involved.

Yet the 4th Session is never ever allowed to be combined along with the 3rd, no matter how urgent and dire the clinical need may seem. In a theoretical case of Sessions 3 and 4 combined, the resulting consent would be considered *invalid*, because of the appearance of a coerced treatment selection made under maximal psychological duress by a patient unable to process and compare the risks and benefits.

The latter is unacceptable from the standpoint of medical ethics. It harkens to the atrocities committed by Nazi "experimenters." Who but they could think of performing "procedures" (both medical and, even worse, surgical) forcibly and against a patient's—or a subject's—will or approval? Of course, no sane colleague in the world today would care to be likened to the brutal criminals spawned by Nazi Germany who notoriously forced patients to undergo treatments under maximal psychological duress!

13.

How to Break Bad News: 4th (Last) Session

The 4th Session Proper

During the 4th Session one informs the patient, in full detail, about specific features or aspects of the various *treatment options* available. These treatment regimens, depending on the patient's diagnosis and prognosis, may be either curative in intent or, if no cure exists, palliative therapies designed to extend life and / or improve quality of life. Any options presented must, of course, be approved therapies indicated for treating a given patient's disease on a case-by-case basis. Then the patient is asked to select one of the indicated treatment regimens available.

The patients need to possess a clear understanding of precisely what to expect from available treatment strategies to be able to determine which is most appropriate for them. Today, cancer treatments often comprise multimodality strategies involving combinations of chemotherapy, radiotherapy, and surgery. Patients need to understand the "expected" *benefits* and *risks* associated with specific treatments. As important, they must understand that "expected" does not mean "guaranteed." Risks including complications, toxicity, mortality, possible loss of an organ or extremity, etc. are always present to varying degrees. Thus, it is exclusively the patient's prerogative—and nobody else's—to weigh all the pros and cons associated with treatment options on those ancient, sacred metaphorical scales entrusted to us by Hippocrates himself, our common Father in the Art of Medicine, who instructed:

Either help or do not harm the patient *

In other words, it is the fully informed patient alone who must decide whether the benefits of a given multimodality strategy outweigh its risks, and either consent to or reject treatment based on his or her own calculations.

---

* Epidemics, Book I, of the Hippocratic school: "Practice two things in your dealings with disease: either help or do not harm the patient". Lloyd GER (1983). Hippocratic Writings, 2nd ed., London 1983: Penguin Books. p. 94.

Neither the physician, nor the relatives, nor anyone else holds this authority.

The patients can only make a qualified decision as to what is best for them if they are fully informed of, and understand, all aspects and parameters involved, without anything hidden or concealed, without deception, without any fine print buried in footnotes of hospital forms, and so on.

Some patients are expected to experience normal human fear that might cause them initially to feel hesitant about accepting aggressive treatments—such as major surgical resection of organs or amputation—that are widely regarded as the best therapeutic options, given the specifics of their case.

Of course, the attending physician has the right to address and clarify any obscure uncertainties in a patient's mind, and attempt to bring him or her back to the real world, while at the same time offering encouraging and comforting words. The doctor reminds the patient that it is cancer they are dealing with—a disease that kills if left untreated. The physician may have to repeat the word 'cancer,' gently, tactfully, but as many times as necessary for the patient to comprehend the gravity of the situation. The patient is encouraged to return to reality, where he or she will be required to make major decisions with a clear head.

The physicians provide responsible advice to a patient who may refuse treatment out of fear; they remind the patient about the inevitable consequences of such a refusal. That is, however, as far as doctors are permitted to go; not an inch farther than reminding and responsibly advising.

No doctor (or anyone else) has the right to make decisions instead of the patients themselves, if the latter are adult and legally sane. The doctor provides advice, information, and points the patient toward the best therapeutic path. Yet the doctor is never entitled to push or pressure patients to choose an unwanted treatment.

We respect our patients' wishes even if we happen to disagree with them. If a patient's wish is utterly irrational, reasons are calmly given that demonstrate why their decision is unreasonable, allowing them to reconsider their position. We also make the patients aware of the consequences of following through with an irrational choice.

We never coerce anyone to undergo any unwanted procedure or treatment, no matter how much we may believe that course is in the patient's best interests. The explanation for this is simple; physicians can only face situations objectively, in an unbiased manner, without calling on subjective intuition, which is considered scientifically unethical. It is only the patients who get to access their spheres of intuition—or even premonition—about their very own being. Wisdom may well exceed the conventional and objective "knowledge" that is based on data gathered by the largest series of patient cases; after all, to a single patient it is only that patient's outcome that matters, not "what is likely to be achieved" on a statistical basis. Ethically, the patients alone are entitled to consider such abstract or philosophical and religious aspects, because doctors are compelled to consider facts and data objectively, based on science only.

Medical ethics is an additional domain that forbids any coercion of patients. Certainly, no doctor in the world would ever wish to be likened to brutal criminals, as explained in the last chapter's end.

Of course, a doctor is not obliged to continue serving as an individual patient's "attending" physician (with full responsibility over the entirety of therapeutic measures) if he or she happens to disagree strongly with this patient's choices. Doctors are never obliged to perform procedures that are contrary to their own medical conscience under any circumstances.

For example, if a patient asks a doctor to amputate an entire upper extremity (all the way down from the axilla or armpit) for a benign small lipoma located in his hand on the grounds of achieving a "radical" resection, then the doctor has no obligation whatsoever to perform a bizarre amputation that is unacceptable and absurd in terms of both common sense and scientific principles. Similarly, a surgeon has no obligation to carry out a pneumonectomy for a small benign hamartoma located at the distal (outer) periphery of the lung. This may be one of the rarer cases, or even a unique case, when a doctor has the right to refuse to continue to accept responsibility for a particular patient's case and he resigns from being "attending." In that case, the resigning doctor proposes another colleague to hand over the case to.

Rarely do matters get so out of hand. It may take a particular patient longer than it usually takes others to make up their minds. And more encouragement and rational explaining may be required to help a patient come to a decision. But almost all patients eventually choose that which is so desired by human nature: the continuance of life, by any means, or even sacrifice.

Fully informed patients do fight more fiercely and more effectively than ill-informed or deceived patients, because the former willingly chose, for example, to sacrifice an organ; the aware patients struggle against their disease with strength, courage, and confidence. We do know how humans are integrated—as a single entity consisting of psyche and body; for this reason, any drop of positive energy (even the smallest droplet) is priceless in empowering the patient to strive to achieve the best possible outcome and continue to persevere fiercely against his illness.

Aware patients do endure postoperative pain, sacrifice, and even some residual disability without a grumble, because they understand in their souls that their very life is at stake.

And now a final word about informing patients when it comes to choosing a particular therapeutic strategy: A universal standard should mandate that attending physician throughout the world be legally obligated to mark holographically each and every patient's folder (or case notes) on the front cover in bold red capital letters stating *Whether* the treatment strategy's goal is *curative intent* and duly sign a statement thereof to that effect, on the basis of staging, fitness, histology, and all other prognostic parameters involved.

That would be the only way for patients to be truly protected from rare, yet potential, *abuse* of their trust in their attending physician. This way they are also protected from potential damage through malice of predatory persons, who may attempt to profit by instilling false hopes in a patient.

The 4th Session: Degree of Comfort

The 4th and last Session of breaking bad news may range from quite comfortable and easy to difficult, uncomfortable, and hard; it all depends on how bad the bad news really is.

(i) Comfortable Sessions

Whenever the stage of a patient's disease happens to be early or the cancer cells' histological type and grade is associated with biological behavior that is less aggressive, significant hope of cure is possible. Most types of thyroid cancers, lymphomas, and early stages (such as "in situ" and "Ia") of epithelial carcinomas may serve as typical examples.

In such cases, breaking the news is easy enough for all: patient, family, informing doctor.

These are the cases with the maximal possible chance of cure, but only if the indicated treatment is appropriately applied. It is easy for the attending doctors to be absolutely frank and encourage their patient to consent to curative treatment. The most effective treatments are usually surgical resection(s) of organ(s) or treatments associated with some degree of toxicity (as chemotherapy offered for treating lymphomas, etc.). It would be a pity for any such patient to remain untreated because he or she may fear the side effects of therapy, when a high probability of cure exists.

Yet nothing can ever be taken for granted, not even obtaining consent from a patient who is likely to be cured; such patients, despite a highly favorable prognosis, may indeed refuse to consent. However, they would likely jump at the opportunity to accept life-saving treatment without having a second thought, if their physician took great care to impress upon them how fortunate they are to have such favorable prognostic factors. It is upon the physician to inform the patient that, all things considered, the bad news isn't really so bad. And it should be especially effective if the physician appears genuinely relieved and optimistic at the findings.

Not surprisingly, therefore, it is generally easier for the doctor to break the bad news to the relatively lucky cancer patients and to also offer fuller and more in-depth information. The doctor needs to do so to encourage the patients to make timely, intelligent decisions that offer realistic hope of being cured.

(ii) Uncomfortable, Difficult Sessions

When disease stage is more advanced or the cancer cell type / grade is aggressive, the chances for a cure can be slim or nonexistent.

In the latter cases, the attending physician who breaks the news faces a disheartening, daunting challenge, for his disclosure route follows a tortuous, thorny path to Golgotha! How much truth can a patient handle, if this person happens to be very sick, desolate, and tired? And even if that patient can indeed handle the truth, will it be of any practical use for him in terms of decision-making, since no cure is expected in his case, regardless of treatment?

In my humble opinion after decades of dealing with humans tormented by cancer, there is no reason to make their experience during Session 4 any more distressing than necessary by extending it in great depth or length at all. In other words, the cancer patient who has no chance for cure should still be informed about the cancer diagnosis of course, yet no full and detailed elaboration on staging and prognosis is recommended, as the latter places an even heavier psychological burden on the person, and that would be of no practical use in terms of choosing among various treatment options.

In such cases, we propose the appropriately indicated treatments only, specifying that these therapies "will *help* them." And the doctor's statement is true, since the treatments will indeed help by either prolonging life or by improving its quality. One needs to remember that the principle aim of disclosure is to help patients make the right therapeutic decisions for a cure; if the latter cannot be achieved, if no curative treatments are available, then there is no reason to upset patients by overloading them more technical details than necessary. If too many unpleasant statistical data on prognosis were offered, we would render them unable to cope with the harsh reality of their situation and, even worse, unable to enjoy and make the best of the time they have left.

Often, these patients subconsciously sense how uncomfortable their doctor feels, hence understand how difficult their own situation is; so, they usually don't ask too many—or excessively detailed—questions. The patient's family members are advised to refrain from asking questions that are awkward, unpleasant, even unintentionally cruel in the presence of the patient.

Let's say that I've just managed to improve a patient's mood a little and finally boost his morale a bit, after having long strived to support and comfort him psychologically.

This hypothetical patient's prognosis is dismal and he has no chance of cure whatsoever because of end-stage disease associated with more unfavorable factors. It would be a devastating blow if a family member were to ask me directly at the conclusion of the consultation "do you mean that …(my husband)… will be cured for sure thanks to the chemotherapy you recommended, doctor?" (Once in my professional life I experienced just such a dreadfully inappropriate direct question by the wife of an unfortunate end–stage patient, after I'd invested a great deal of time comforting and offering support to the poor man.)

There's also an article* published in 'The Guardian' about the *fearful* difficulty doctors face, whenever they have to break such unpalatable news to patients.

During this final session, the doctors still have no right to lie, yet on rare occasions they may be forced to disclose only a substantial part of the truth, but not the whole truth. In the most uncomfortable cases in which the truth is

---

* Jalal Baig. *Facing my fear: telling a cancer patient he was going to die.* The Guardian, May 27, 2016:
    https://www.theguardian.com/commentisfree/2016/may/27/facing-my-fear-telling-cancer-patient-terminal-illness-diagnosis

exceedingly grim, it is the doctors' clinical experience, or wisdom, that guides them to determine how much of the truth a given patient can handle while receiving the news.

Even in the hardest cases, though, physicians are compelled to verbally disclose something about the "difficulty of treating that particular case being relatively greater" or about "the prognosis being somewhat less favorable" than in other cases. The physicians are obliged to deliver the disclosure with empathy and nonverbal gestures and postures of concerned persons, to protect their patient from exploitation at the hands of certain cunning professionals, who would attempt to profit by offering false hopes to vulnerable patients for whom no cures exist.

14.

Documentation, Staging, Treatments

Clinical Counterexample

An elderly man named Constantine had to be hospitalized, one cold winter's night, due to a high fever. The fever, as it turned out, was caused by a relatively benign viral infection. Unfortunately, because his past medical history was incomplete, contained inaccurate information, and Constantine had a poor understanding of his true history, the attending physicians were unable to determine the correct diagnosis.

On x-ray, the entire right side of Constantine's chest appeared to be so thoroughly congested with fluid that the lung itself couldn't be seen. A distinctive scar on the right side of the chest indicated that a thoracotomy had been performed at some time in the patient's past. Thoracotomy is a surgical procedure that opens the chest permitting access to the heart, lungs, esophagus, etc. Unfortunately, specific information regarding the exact nature of Constantine's thoracotomy was unavailable. Moreover, the patient himself was unsure about significant details regarding his medical history. All Constantine could recall and report was that eighteen years prior, he had undergone what he understood to be a "minor, standard" surgical procedure involving his right lung, and the thoracic surgeon who performed it had long since passed away. The junior physicians on call mistakenly assumed the patient's prior procedure involved nothing more than an open lung biopsy or, perhaps, a plain wedge resection.

Constantine carried with him an enormous plastic bag filled with laboratory test results dating from his hospital admission those many years ago. Most of the old results no longer held any diagnostic value. But among the myriad outdated documents was an old hand-typed histopathology report; it was succinct, to say the least, stating only that the surgical specimen was "negative for malignancy." The report didn't even provide a macroscopic description of the specimen examined, but it did bear the coded capital

Roman letter *"F"* in addition to a long numerical value in its *"our reference"* field.

In years past, the Roman upper-case *"F"* was used in Greece as a code to alert clinicians that the histopathology results reported on that document were intentionally *falsified* to set the patient's mind at ease and instill an unwarranted sense of relief. Physicians of that era knew well that they should ignore results reported on an *F*-marked report, which was issued solely for the patient's *"benefit,"* and that the actual results would be positive for malignancy. The old practice of lying in writing has been abandoned in modern Greece. As such, contemporary physicians are generally unaware that older reports marked *"F"* contain false information that should be ignored. Accordingly, the junior physicians on call when Constantine presented were misled by the same bogus results intended long ago to mislead their patient and had no reason to suspect that he underwent pneumonectomy to remove a cancerous lung—they did not have access to relevant data.

Constantine's wife had also died since his surgery, and she carried the secret of his cancer and pneumonectomy (removal of an entire lung) to her *grave. The procedure was successful and Constantine was cured, but he was never informed by anyone that he had cancer and that his right lung was removed. His lung couldn't be seen on current x-ray films because it had been removed 18 years prior.*

Lacking this critical information, the on-call specialist-trainees mistakenly, but understandably (given the circumstances) diagnosed a large pleural effusion (accumulation of fluid) of infectious origin that was compressing the lung. They repeatedly tapped the effusion, attempting to evacuate the fluid, which would allow the (unbeknownst to them, missing) lung to expand. They even inserted catheters inside the chest to facilitate evacuation and achieve pulmonary expansion. In fact, the presence of fluid was normal. Immediately after pneumonectomy, the empty space left by the resected lung is filled with air, which is then gradually replaced by fluid. It's a predictable change following this procedure. Unfortunately for Constantine, the post-pneumonectomy space became infected due to multiple insertions of needles and catheters. Infection is always a risk, despite careful attention to meticulous aseptic techniques.

Constantine survived lung cancer and lived his first 18 postoperative years reasonably well, but suddenly that would all change. Complications from the treatment he received after misdiagnosis led to iatrogenic (caused by medical examination or treatment) post-pneumonectomy empyema thoracis. Constantine would suffer the unpleasant consequences of this condition for the rest of his life.

The empyema surely would have been avoided if Constantine had been aware of the pneumonectomy or if the treating physicians had access to adequate **documentation** of that procedure (an authentic, official Operative Record, for example).

Lies survived truth, and Constantine suffered needlessly, because two people—his wife and his surgeon—took to their graves the secret of his cancer and how it was treated. Consequently, the clinicians treating Constantine were deprived of critical information they needed to know that would have saved much precious time and spared their patient unnecessary immediate and long-term suffering.

"Garbage in, garbage out" is a popular aphorism used by people who work in fields such as computer science, mathematics, information technology, and similar fields rooted in analysis and logic. It's used to express the idea that flawed input (garbage in) will always produce flawed output (garbage out) in systems that depend on logical processes. The case reported above clearly demonstrates how it also applies in medical decision-making processes. The young physicians trying to make an accurate diagnosis using the flawed information available to them unwittingly produced highly flawed results. Had they access to accurate records and a true history, one could reasonably expect that Constantine would have enjoyed a favorable outcome.

Medical Documentation

All accurate aspects, technical details and parameters regarding patients' diseases, their surgical procedures, in-hospital admissions and discharges, as well as their past medical history must be precisely recorded or documented, provided they have been proven.

Any parameters of relatively higher significance or importance than others must be annotated and underlined for emphasis during their documentation or recording inside the patient's files. This attention to emphasizing, or "flagging," important items eliminates the risk of their being concealed or lost in an ocean of data of lesser significance*.

I'm afraid that in Greece and certain other countries, when one attends an outpatients' clinic for an appointment, one is usually seen carrying around a huge envelope filled with smaller envelopes of various sizes filled with test results, thrown inside haphazardly without any thought given to order (either by clinical significance, chronology, or

---

* Please, see the same author's ebook *"Differential Clinical Significance of Medical Information,"* Thessaloniki 2016: www.papachristos.eu/dcsmi

otherwise). A comprehensive medical report is rarely provided. But one should be, and it ought to include all clinically significant health parameters, recorded in an orderly way, along with any laboratory test results that are remarkable or important.

In the hospitals of some countries, such as Greece, a blank new patient record folder is opened when a patient is admitted or readmitted—every single time. Information from previous admissions is not transferred to the new folder. Thus, the quantity of information yielded from previous admissions is incrementally lost to history. The patients themselves rarely recall precise diagnoses from their past histories and struggle to recall them when a new medical history is taken with each new admission. The data lost may be valuable or determinatively significant; they may have been painstakingly documented after invasive procedures of great cost and risk to the patient.

Often, in some countries, patients' case notes may even be patchy and deficient, lacking a recorded clinical history or documentation of other clinical information. Some patients' case files contain nothing more than reports of laboratory results with no records of other significant information, such as past history, medications, physical-examination findings, etc.

In the UK, on the other hand, and in other developed countries, previous in-patients' case notes are maintained in the hospital's archives and retrieved whenever a patient is re-admitted to the same hospital for any reason. New pages are added to this single set of case notes as new information accumulates and is recorded. The patient's record is, thus, cumulative; new information is added to previous records, which will contain older reports of the patient's history, physical examination findings, laboratory test results, and other entries dating from the patient's first encounter. This is a time saver for busy junior physicians, as they only need to update the most recent section of the patient's history: older facts and data are current up to his previous hospital stay.

If a physician is reproached for failure to produce well-written, comprehensive medical reports and case notes, the usual excuse offered is that he attempted "to avoid accidental disclosure of the cancer diagnosis" should the patient happen to read the documents. Yet it's reasonable to suspect that the real reason is an indifferent, off-handed, careless attitude in general (coupled with laziness and sloth) as well as a deliberate "strategy of minimal effort" (a cynical work ethic adopted perhaps by busy, yet *underpaid*, staff in poor countries), along with a pure lack of professionalism.

Humane physicians who endeavor to avoid upsetting cancer patients with unpleasant diagnoses in Greece and elsewhere could make a greater contribution by actively promoting and enforcing the introduction of proper medical documentation principles; such principles will greatly benefit the patients concerned.

Staging

After cancer is diagnosed, the next important process, as it applies to making treatment decisions, is disease staging. When this process is completed, a given patient's stage is signified by a capital Roman numeral, usually from one (I) up to four (IV). The precise numbers may vary, depending on the type of cancer.

For some cancers, "sub-stages" are also used, and they are likewise labelled using Roman letters, usually in lower case (a, b, c, and so on), after the capital Roman number of the main stage.

For instance, there are four main stages of lung cancer: I, II, III, and IV. Yet there are nine sub-stages of lung cancer: Ia, Ib, IIa, IIb, IIIa, IIIb, IIIc, IVa, IVb (moving from early to later or more-advanced stages.)

A "T N M" staging system is also in use. The abbreviated letters come from **T**umor, **N**ode (lymph-node involvement), and the presence or lack of **M**etastases. Numerical values (or "descriptors") are applied to each of the

TNM letters; so, a cancer may be staged as:

- T0 or Tx or T1 or T2 or T3 or T4, and
- N0 or N1 or N2 or N3, and
- M0 or M1.

Tables have been developed that accurately convert any given combination of TNM descriptors into a certain stage grouping. In lung cancer, for instance, T3 N1 M0 is assigned to stage IIIa (or the IIIa grouping of stage).

Recent staging revisions include the introduction of further sub-groupings for each sub-stage (a given sub-stage may be further divided into yet more subordinate stages). For instance, according to the 8th revision of staging lung cancer, three subordinate stages are found within the Ia substage (Ia$_1$, Ia$_2$, and Ia$_3$).

Staging is extremely significant because it is used to determine treatment strategies and which modalities ought to be applied (for instance surgical or nonsurgical treatment), but it is also useful in determining prognosis and other parameters.

The details of exactly how to stage various kinds of cancer (and similar malignant diseases) accurately are established on an international scale by prestigious professional organizations or scientific societies such as the NCCN (National Comprehensive Cancer Network, www.nccn.org). In addition, scientific societies that focus on specific cancers also contribute to the development of staging guidelines; in lung cancer, for instance, the IASLC (International Association for the Study of Lung Cancer, www.iaslc.org) is involved.

These organizations study enormous patient populations, with varying disease characteristics, so they are able to reach conclusions on methods of staging that are statistically significant for purposes of prognosis as well as for choosing treatments, etc. Every system is usually subject to regular revisions and improvements, so that new data are periodically reviewed with the aim of improving accuracy in proper staging.

Any in-depth elaboration on concepts in staging is beyond the scope of this book. Some general principles, however, need to be clarified to protect patients from what I term *"Commercialization of forlorn hopes"* (or the attempts of unethical professionals to profit financially by deliberately offering forlorn hopes to patients with advanced disease).

Cancer arises from a single mutated cell. This cell rapidly proliferates by dividing uncontrollably; it does so at the expense of adjacent healthy, normal cells and tissues. The cancer cells often invade or "infiltrate" normal surrounding cells, which destroys healthy tissue. The size of the cancer, or tumor, usually grows larger relatively fast. Its stage is considered "early," as long as the tumor is still confined to the organ in which it initially developed—the "primary site." The larger the tumor, of course, the higher and more advanced its stage.

There comes a critical moment when the cancer reaches the outer limits of the primary organ. From there the tumor may extend beyond the initial disease site and invade adjacent tissues or organs. Such *contiguous* invasion means the disease stage has progressed to "intermediate," i.e., a somewhat more advanced stage. There is still hope of achieving a cure, even at this intermediate stage, albeit the odds are slightly reduced.

If unchecked, sooner or later the tumor reaches and invades adjacent vessels (e.g., lymphatic or blood). Cancer cells then travel via circulation in these vessels and disseminate to distant sites or regions of the body. That's what one means by saying "disease *spread*." There are two distinct routes of circulatory dissemination; "lymphatic spread" (via lymph nodes or lymph glands and lymphoid tissues) and "hematogenous (or blood-borne) spread." Cancerous cells disseminated via these routes can cause "distant metastases" or "secondary deposits" of the disease. They attack organs or tissues that are *not* in anatomical contact with the site of origin.

These "distant metastases" can be located in any site throughout the body. Yet they are more often found in organs and tissues that receive a substantially large amount of blood flow through vessels of rather narrow lumen, such as the liver, the lungs, the brain, the adrenal glands, the spleen, the skin etc.

Throughout the world, *staging* is understood as the attempted unbiased, *meticulous* assessment of the existing stage in a particular cancer of a given patient on the basis of hard evidence provided by systemic, thorough, extensive, and *exhaustive* search for any evidence of disease dissemination in the body. Assumption that a cancer is contained within the organ in which it initially arose is *not* allowed, instead it is necessary to *prove* either the absence or the presence of any spread to distant sites in the patient's body. Even the particular details of the cancer's local extension (size or dimensions of the primary tumor reaching or not the outer limits of the primary organ, possible breaching of those limits, possible invasion of surrounding or adjacent tissues, etc.) need to be precisely documented and recorded. Cancer staging, thus, is the process of determining the nature and extent of disease.

Conventional staging techniques usually include Computed Tomography or CT scanning of the chest, abdomen, and brain, bone scintigraphy (or "bone scanning" with ^{99m}Tc or other radioisotopes), as well as more specific laboratory investigations, depending on the cancer type and location (i.e., in lung cancer of the left upper lobe an additional laryngoscopy is necessary; in esophageal cancer, an additional bronchoscopy is needed, and so on). Staging isn't always based on laboratory investigations alone, but clinical examinations as well (palpation to detect any enlarged or swollen lymph nodes, a possible enlargement of liver or spleen, a possible endoscopy examination, etc.).

In the modern era, staging has benefited by achieving greater accuracy from the use of Positron Emission Tomography scanning in conjunction with CT (PET / CT). The latter is the *best available* and most effective tool to detect and reveal distant metastases or lymphatic spread, and it is considered substantially superior to conventional staging.

There should be no doubt that thorough, meticulous, and exhaustive staging has been completed *before* one is allowed to consider and discuss which treatments are appropriate for a given patient's particular case. Any violation of this principle may lead to catastrophic consequences; it can result in a patient receiving suboptimal or contraindicated treatment for his disease type and stage.

Early stages are defined by cancer contained within the primary organ site, without any extension (neither to the outer limits of that organ nor outside of it). Spread of the disease, or metastasis, elsewhere in the body must be absent.

Intermediate stages are defined by cancer reaching the outer limits of the initial organ or, worse, by breaching those limits and extending into adjacent tissues or organs. In the latter case, cancer must still be contained within some wider particular anatomical region. The infiltrated adjacent tissues or organs cannot be considered "vital"; i.e., they must be considered "resectable," able to be safely removed in those stages*. Disease is then considered

---

* If, for example, the heart, aorta, or similarly vital, non-removable organs are invaded, then the stage no longer qualifies as "intermediate."

more advanced. In intermediate stages, there should be *no* distant spread of the disease elsewhere in the body.

Advanced stages of cancer are defined by either contiguous (direct) extension of tumor into an adjacent *vital* organ (e.g., the heart, etc.) or by *spread* of the disease into either distant sites or into (more or less remote) lymph nodes or lymph glands. For staging purposes, one tends to consider the presence or absence of spread as a "Qualitative only" feature; in other words, as either "true" or "false" (spread either exists or it doesn't), but not as a "quantitative" feature of cancer. If there is spread documented, then a case is staged as advanced (by degrees), no matter how great or small the actual number of distant metastases is. Needless to say, a patient is better off without any spread.

The presence of spread is always ominous, but its clinical significance varies according to degree; it can be "less worrisome" (e.g., lymphatic spread to local or regional or neighboring lymph glands only, with absence of distant metastases) or "more worrisome" (blood-borne dissemination or spread to multiple distant sites).

Some unscrupulous physicians have been suspected of *deliberately* ordering **incomplete** studies, *omitting* requests for tests specifically designed to detect disease dissemination in their patients. As a result, an unfortunate patient's disease may well have spread, yet remain undetected because the proper investigations were deliberately *not* requested. For example, if brain CT scanning is not requested, then any brain metastases present will, of course, go undetected. Thus, it would appear on paper that a patient's lung cancer, for example, is contained within the lung, and that the disease is still at an early stage. How could such a travesty be permitted? A physician who would stoop to such heartless, unethical subterfuge is motivated by pure greed. A patient diagnosed with early-stage disease can be convinced by an aggressive, persuasive physician to undergo the most expensive forms of anticancer treatment...treatment, incidentally, that would be inappropriate and contraindicated in persons with advanced-stage disease. The more expensive the treatment, the greater the financial benefit for the physician.

In other words, there is some concern that a few corrupt professionals may be exploiting unfortunate patients by deliberate and intentional omission of complete and meticulous staging procedures, so that any existing dissemination remains undetected, undiagnosed, and unknown. The physician then persuades the patients that expensive major surgery, contraindicated in advanced disease, is their best option. Such unfathomable *exploitation* might well take place not only in poor countries, such as Greece, but also in wealthy countries with a predominantly *private* healthcare system in place. The exorbitant fees billed to private patients may act as the tempting motive for a handful of dishonest, unethical physicians.

Treatments

The various ways of treating cancer can be grouped into two main categories:

A. *Regional or Local (Loco-regional) Treatments:*

    i. <u>Complete surgical resection of an entire organ:</u> This involves resection (removal) of the whole organ in which the primary cancer developed. For instance, resection of a pulmonary lobe or of the uterus (womb), or breast, or larynx (voice box), or of a testicle, and so on. A similar concept exists; that of a wider (or "radical") major resection. The latter is the removal of an entire organ along with simultaneous removal of surrounding tissues (or parts of adjacent organs) that are found directly infiltrated by a rather limited extension of cancer during surgery. Such resections are performed whenever and *if* there is *curative* intent; they are considered by far *the most effective* ways of treating cancer in order to achieve a cure, but *only if* the initial indication for carrying them out was correct and properly set in the first place.

ii. <u>Surgical resection of the tumor alone</u> with resection margins negative for disease: This describes a more limited resection, during which the surgeons attempt to resect also surrounding healthy-appearing tissues in order to remove a surgical specimen with adequately wide margins of cancer-free tissues around the resected primary tumor. Guidelines exist regarding the minimal dimensions that must exist between the outer limits of the tumor and the resection margins for it to be considered safe (usually in the range of 2.5 – 5 cm). Such limited, "non-radical" resections are considered *"less effective"* in achieving a cure; they are, however, therapeutically useful in certain cases for cytoreduction, subject to the patients' attending physicians' recommendation. These procedures are also known as *"excisional* biopsies."

iii. <u>Radiotherapy:</u> administered either via external irradiation targeted to reach deeply located organs or tissues while sparing surrounding healthy tissue, or "brachytherapy," the implantation of radioactive seeds or similar materials into a tumor to destroy it locally. It can also be offered for prevention purposes into regions of the body, such as the brain, into which chemotherapy drugs cannot readily penetrate. Radiotherapy *can* achieve cures and is generally considered less risky than surgical treatment. Yet the effectiveness of radiotherapy alone may well be lesser than resection.

iv. <u>Local ablation</u> of the tumor, usually thermal ablation, achieved by various techniques (diathermy, radiofrequency, LASER, CyberKnife, and similar *palliative* methods). In clinical practice, one uses ablation as part of a wider therapeutic set, or "package," along with additional therapeutic techniques involved in a multimodality treatment strategy.

B. Systemic or Generalized Treatments:

i. <u>Chemotherapy:</u> Simultaneous administration of drugs (usually by intravenous infusions, but sometimes orally, too, in the form of pills), which enter the bloodstream wherein they circulate throughout the body, with the aim of killing or destroying cancer cells, wherever the latter are encountered. These drugs usually can't penetrate into the patients' brains, as they're blocked by the blood-brain barrier. Chemotherapy drugs often damage healthy cells, too (especially rapidly multiplying normal cells); thus, the body needs time to recover after each course of chemotherapy. Accordingly, chemotherapy is usually administered in "*cycles;*" first, there's the simultaneous administration of some chemotherapy drugs over one or two days, followed by an interval of typically 3 – 4 weeks off-treatment recovery time. After the preset drug-free interval, another chemotherapy cycle is administered, and so on. Chemotherapy is often associated with undesirable treatment-emergent adverse effects, such as nausea and vomiting, fatigue, hair loss, etc., which are usually transient and fully reversible.

ii.   Newer systemic treatments are expected to emerge in the future based on ongoing research. Research has thus far revealed promising results with agents that act with the patient's immune system; indeed, primitive immunotherapy regimens and vaccines exist that seem to hold some promise.

People are often with the impression that surgery offers the best hope for cure in cancer cases in general. That understanding is reasonable indeed, but only when circumstances permit. In other words, that statement is *only valid if* surgery was employed to treat a patient's disease whose stage was either "early," or "limited," or in any case "contained" (within an organ or a single anatomical region that can be safely removed surgically). To clarify further, the absence of any spread of cancer *must have first been proven* for any kind of loco-regional treatment to be indicated, either with surgery or radiotherapy.

For instance, let's consider a tree affected by some sort of generalized disease, diffusely disseminated all over: apparent on the trunk, but also in many of the branches, with roots rotten and so on. A tree surgeon cannot possibly save this tree by chopping off the many affected parts; even if one were to try to do so, the tree couldn't survive after undergoing too many multiple amputations. This unfortunate tree's only viable hope is the administration of an appropriate "medication" (pesticide, perhaps) administered by an arborist; then the drug may well stimulate circulation in the sap "stream" of the tree, combatting the disseminated, generalized illness throughout.

Similarly, patients with disseminated cancer in miscellaneous regions or distant organs require a generalized form of treatment, such as chemotherapy, that acts throughout the body's system. Treating these patients' cancer with loco-regional methods (such as surgery) is definitely not going to result in a cure, no matter how skillfully a surgeon may resect the primary tumor; even with radical surgical resection, viable cancer cells will remain in each remote metastatic site after the procedure. Hence, these patients will not emerge cancer-free. Not even a single cancer cell can remain viable at the end of any surgical procedure for it to be considered "curative." Otherwise, it's merely an *"incomplete"* resection that cannot, unfortunately, lead to cure!

Patients must also be *fit* for surgery. In other words, their general state of health must allow a reasonable chance of their withstanding the surgery and surviving it. Physicians often have to make unbiased decisions about their patients' fitness (or unfitness) on the grounds of objectively calculated risks; for instance, reserves of respiratory function can be accurately quantified, in order to compute the "predicted postoperative" respiratory function of a particular patient post pneumonectomy, prior to performing that major resection. In plain words, if the capacity of the postoperative remaining lung is adequate for the continuation of a patient's life, only then can one perform the procedure.

In philosophy as well as in real life, every benefit always comes at some cost or with some risk. Similarly, in physics the *entropy* of any given system always tends to increase; hence energy must be provided for some essential order to remain somewhere to avert chaos and disorder.

Similarly, there's unfortunately and inevitably *a double price to pay* in treating cancer with surgery. First, an organ is usually resected (removed) or an extremity is amputated; in other words, there's some *sacrifice*. Second, each and every medical or surgical procedure (even the most minor one) is always associated with inherent *risks* of both mortality and morbidity, which never equal zero in any setting or place in the world.

Of course, at this point of the book I must note that surgical resection of *deeply located internal* vital organs does usually carry significant mortality risks (as such are considered risks within the range of 5%, 7%, 10%, 15%, and so on). One refers to such resections as major surgery.

On the contrary, everything is easier, from the purely technical point of view, at least, in resections of organs that are not vital (aren't necessary for the continuation of one's life) or which are easily accessible, *externally located* structures. For instance, women's breasts and men's testicles both may well hold a high value in emotional, psychological, ethical, or literary terms, yet their resection is technically relatively simple and straightforward, since the surgeon need not open the body to access these structures (as with thoracotomy to access the lung to perform pneumonectomy). So, surgical risks are quite low compared with the risks inherent in, say, a pancreatic resection.

The above-mentioned realities offer an explanation for clinically justifying the use of surgical treatment on the basis of "wider" or more "relative" or more "relaxed" indications, if the organ to be sacrificed happens to be "easy to resect" (i.e., either externally located or resectable with minimal risks).

Yet the mere fact that "a tumor is resectable" does not qualify as a proper indication for using surgery under any circumstances or pretexts whatsoever. A true *indication* for treating cancer with surgery only exists if all three of the following criteria are met: (a) no dissemination of the disease was detected after full and meticulous evaluation, (b) the patient must be fit enough to withstand and survive the surgery on the basis of objective assessments, and (c) the tumor must, of course, be resectable in the first place.

Of course, nowadays *multimodality* treatment—the combination of more than one method of treatment together, or in a predefined consecutive series—is employed more and more often. One usually strives to increase the overall effectiveness of the therapy this way.

Whenever, for instance, the cancer stage is somewhat advanced (but not "too advanced"), one may achieve "down staging" by administering "induction treatment" ("neoadjuvant" treatment). Afterwards, depending on the results of induction treatment, successful surgical resection with curative intent may be feasible.

In other cases, complementary radiotherapy may be needed postoperatively, for instance, at the mediastinum (the middle most inner part of the chest), or adjuvant chemotherapy for maximizing the therapeutic results (improving the statistical possibility of achieving a cure).

Nowadays, therapeutic options do exist and can usually be employed even in rather unfavorable and difficult cases, on the condition that the enacted-as-valid indications are honestly respected (correctly applied); i.e., without subterfuge or deceit.

15.

Preparing Families When the End Draws Near: Caution

Clinical Counterexample

In a somber hospital room, an unfortunate middle-aged woman lay moribund, languishing in excruciating pain. Cancer had invaded all her pelvic organs, causing a condition known as "frozen pelvis." Her body was essentially divided into two parts at the pelvis. Her condition was so severe that the flow of blood, urine, and other bodily fluids and the transmission of neural impulses and stimuli between her upper and lower body became a source of agonizing, unbearable pain.

Her family members had, of course, been informed of the cancer diagnosis, but the details of her condition were described using highly technical, esoteric medical terminology. Accordingly, her unfortunate relatives were understandably confused and did not understand that their loved one had incurable terminal disease; death was imminent and the poor woman's suffering would soon end.

The alarmed, highly agitated relatives were pacing up and down the corridors of the large, state-owned hospital in Thessaloniki (Greece's second-largest city) desperately looking for a savior to rescue the patient. Whenever her potassium level became dangerously low, they pressured any physician they could find—an internist, or even an endocrinologist—to bring it back into the normal range. Anytime the patient went into tachycardia (an abnormally fast heart rate) they did everything in their power to ensure that a cardiologist would immediately appear at her bedside, in the mistaken belief that the woman's life could be saved. They really couldn't be blamed for being so aggressive; they were left with the false impression that the patient could be saved provided her potassium levels were properly regulated, that her arrhythmias were corrected, and any other abnormal developments were attended to and kept under control.

The attending physicians were, of course, to blame for the whole mess. They should have explained clearly to the family that the patient's cancer was by then so far advanced and so widely disseminated that nothing could be done to stop the inevitable. Every vital function was failing; systems were shutting down one after another in a cascade-like manner, and death was imminent. Her suffering would soon end, and she would at last be at peace.

The patient had the right to receive palliative care, to be treated with respect, to maintain her dignity, and to live as comfortably as possible during her most precious remaining moments during the terminal phase of her disease. Proper hydration and optimal administration of opiates—potent painkillers that also relieve the anxiety associated with imminent death—would have been the best course of action for this patient.

Instead, she was surrounded by frightened, panicked family members so desperate to save her that they actually grappled with the idea of seeking out potential acquaintances of high-ranking government officials (e.g., Members of Parliament, Cabinet Members, or any high-ranking influential figures) to act as liaisons on her behalf. They hoped to find people connected in any way to powerful government officials *who might be persuaded to use their considerable influence to pressure hospital administrative officials into providing more medical experts and resources, whatever it might take, to save their relative. The family believed that if the patient were surrounded by an array of diverse specialists, it would be possible to stabilize her vital functions, which continued to fail, one after another. The whole scene resembled an unseemly circus, an appallingly sad spectacle playing out under tragic circumstances.*

The dying patient's ordeal lasted for four whole days and nights. The family members' ordeal lasted just as long, except their misery derived from a sense of helplessness and all-consuming feelings of guilt. They felt personally responsible for ensuring that everything possible was being done to maintain the patient's potassium level in the normal range. As if maintaining normal electrolyte levels would miraculously eliminate the cancer, which by then was so advanced, it virtually dammed up the organs of her pelvis, effectively partitioning her body into two unsustainable portions that could not survive.

Continuation of Chapter 15

Due caution should always be exercised by all caregivers when it comes to cancer and providing information. One must consider the cancer patients themselves on one hand, and their family members on the other. As compassionate human beings, we feel a need to paint the brightest picture, to accentuate the positive and maximize patients' hopes and expectations that they might not become disconsolate, fearful, or anxious about their condition. This approach, however, is inappropriate when it comes to dealing with family members or other close relatives.

If a physician should decide that it is prudent to omit, for the moment, a particularly bitter portion of the truth while informing a given patient, the same physician is obligated to reveal all—the unadorned whole truth, no matter how unpleasant or frightening—when informing the family. This is necessary because physicians are obligated to prepare close relatives emotionally and protect them from the potential psychological damage of guilt syndromes, as illustrated in the above Counterexample.

The family members—if left unaware of how dismal, or terminal, the prognosis is—will instinctively and aggressively do whatever they feel it takes to preserve the life of their own flesh and blood. They will, by any means possible, attempt to achieve what unknown to them, is truly impossible.

Hence, frightened family members often panic and act out in desperation; they may become aggressive and / or belligerent toward staff. They come to believe the patient isn't receiving the care and attention they need. They become frustrated during times when minimal on-call staff are present due to, for example, bank holidays. They complain about the lack of highly specialized medical experts (whose involvement would do nothing to stop or forestall imminent death) or about the shortage or unavailability of expensive medication. They take matters into their own hands and try to find ways to get things accomplished through outside channels, such as actively searching out "intermediary politicians" to pull strings and exert influence. Desperate people will understandably resort to all manner of extreme schemes if they're allowed to harbor false hopes that their loved one—their own flesh and blood—can still be saved.

Moreover, after an inevitable death, the family may even pursue litigation for alleged malpractice, as if physicians can be held medically negligent for failing to perform a miracle.

Consider the case of an unfortunate woman who died of breast cancer after nine years of various therapeutic maneuvers. The patient exceeded the expected "life expectancy" according to the literature regarding her disease; yet, her relatives displayed ingratitude. Instead of being happy for the quite significant life extension enjoyed by the patient, they began engaging in accusations and legal disputes for pecuniary compensation!

Did any physician by chance guarantee the relatives that their loved one would live eternally…for ever and ever? Or did they themselves misconstrue, according to their own liking, the somewhat dissimilar disclosure statement offered by some physician? Was the latter, by chance, not clear enough or not realistic enough—as well as ominous enough—as he ought to have been?

As a consequence, some physicians stood unjustly accused, were slandered and subjected to awkward and embarrassing legal defense aggravations. Perhaps some overly-optimistic, unreal, or even mystical notions had gone to the accusers' heads. Such notions might indeed have been suggested by an irresponsible "Dr. Addlebrain."

This "Dr. Addlebrain" didn't need to spend any time at all offering encouragement or psychological support. He didn't have to endure (for long) any crying nor did he wipe off any teardrops. He presumed that he could possibly get away with merely promising the moon (and the earth, too) to the patients' relatives, saving time by instantly making them happy and smiling: no crystal-clear disclosure about the dismal prognosis, no warning about the imminent death, relatives made happy for a while, resulting in no time wasted of his own at all. Despite everybody's initial joy, the final, sad outcome did occur after all; this result made the unwarned and unprepared relatives cry even harder, sob, and endlessly weep. However, in the end, "Dr. Addlebrain" also cried, when he found himself standing in the dock.

Of course, a preexisting psychiatric disorder—depression, personality disorder, etc.—may afflict one or more of the grieving relatives, for they too are only human. Still, it is almost always the case that a thoughtless attending physician is to blame for the panicky relatives' erratic behavior: the relatives ought to have been informed and prepared to deal with the imminent death of their loved one, but that derelict physician neglected to do so.

There may be, unfortunately, some colleagues who like to be "exclusively pleasant only," and nothing else but that to both patients and their relatives. They even try hard to sound casual or be playful as if they were candidates for municipal or parliamentary elections. Some other colleagues simply can't cope with having to break bad news; the latter should definitely not practice their profession—on a clinical basis, at least—or they should request a psychiatrist's assistance for themselves.

The medical profession requires us to break bad news, too, whenever there is some to be broken, regardless of whether we want to or not. Failure to fulfill that requirement results in catastrophes similar to the ones mentioned above, and worse.

The utmost caution is required, when one at once breaks bad news while trying to offer some comfort, hope, and encouragement. The hope offered must be somewhat realistic, taking into account the precise features of a given case and tailored for the needs unique to the case. Offering overly optimistic, unrealistic, and far-fetched hope is strictly forbidden.

It is the closest members of the family who specifically need to be warned when death is imminent, so that they may prepare themselves for the approaching cataclysm, an emotional upheaval that could profoundly assault the foundations of their own being with waves of guilt. The approaching, inevitable outcome must be explained to the family members unequivocally using a short, simple phrase that leaves no room for doubt in anyone's heart. The words are dark, poignant, as painful to speak as they are to hear, and as final as the grave. They must be told that the patient, their own flesh and blood, *"...is dying."*

So yes, we do offer hope and comfort, but reasonably so—in moderation and with a sense of realism. As just discussed, we must also inform the closest family members when the end draws near. They need to understand that death will come, one way or another— whether the mode be cardiac arrest, respiratory failure, coma, etc.—despite our fiercest, and inexorably futile, efforts to defeat it and keep inevitably failing systems functioning. In other words, in such cases death will come even without our permission.

When malignant disease reaches a terminal stage, it exhausts the body's ability to defend itself and maintain life. It leads to an overwhelming series of rapidly occurring catastrophic events, much like a chain reaction; each and every event is by itself potentially fatal. These events include hyper–calcemia, hyper– or hypo–kalemia, hypo– or hyper- natremia, cardiac arrhythmia (severe disturbance in heart rhythm), severe arterial hypotension (extremely low blood pressure; aka "shock"), respiratory failure, renal failure, multi-organ failure, and so forth.

This domino effect of death resembles the quandary of defeating the legendary *Lernaean Hydra**. The Hydra had nine (or more) heads; every time someone attempting to slay the beast would cut off one head, two more would grow out of the stump. It was a hopeless task, unless you were Hercules. Similarly, each time we treat one potentially fatal event, others continue to emerge, and thus the cycle will continue until the patient dies. All we manage to accomplish with this approach is to prolong the agony of a moribund patient who cannot be saved.

Caution is once again needed here. Patients themselves are the main focus of attention, not their relatives. The patients are entitled not to be tormented during their

---

* The Lernaean Hydra was a water-snake–like monster in Greek mythology. It had nine (or more) heads and every time someone would cut off one of them, two more heads would grow out of the stump. The slaying of it was one of Hercules's "Twelve Labors." Hercules cauterized the stump of each severed head until he finally slain the immortal head, too, of the monster. The term is herein used in the meaning of a multifarious and difficult situation.

precious, most sacrosanct moments before death. They are undeniably entitled to a humane death. In some countries things are so poorly regulated (or not regulated at all) in these matters that they seem absurd. Greece seems to be one of them, probably as a remnant of a four-centuries–long Turkish Ottoman occupation (resulting in some subservience) and of another couple centuries of absurdity and corruption (imposed by the many degenerated ruling structures of the modern Greek state). What can physicians actively do to safeguard a patient's right to a humane death while at the same time remaining within the limits of the law when faced with totally unregulated or poorly regulated mandates regarding medical decisions and interventions at life's end?

Both in the remote past and recently, I witnessed cardiopulmonary resuscitation attempted in a patient with end-stage cancer. For what purpose? It was an *appalling and absurd* idea, whose memories still haunt me today. How could it be of any benefit whatsoever for the unfortunate patient to be revived into a state of ongoing suffering from terminal-stage cancer, then having to be submitted again to the very same ordeal of dying for a second time? What for?

If dying is considered a traumatic experience, then how humane is it for physicians to compel cancer patients to die again, for a second time (and then maybe a third or fourth time, and so on), after a "successful" resuscitation, after having already actively experienced the dying process once? That is a profoundly important question, to be dealt with in the chapters that follow.

In the present chapter I deliberately referred to the patient's relatives, instead of referring to the patients themselves, for—in many countries such as Greece—the family members always are physically present at the dying patients' bedside, thus influencing their mood. I referred to the caution that is due while providing information to the relatives: we have the duty to keep them updated with the patient's real situation, no matter how dismal that is. Exposing the relatives to some sad realities is, alas, the only practical way to help them psychologically, meaning that then they will be *prepared* to face the unavoidable sequence of their loved one's inevitable death.

This is also the only feasible way to achieve the relatives' collaboration with the nursing staff without any guilty panic of their own, in preparation for safeguarding the moribund patients' certain humane end with dignity, respect, calmness, and comfort.

The reason I dealt herein with relatives is that it is they who affect the patients most during their most sacrosanct time, defined by a great need for humanness, support, and love!

16.

How Much of The Truth

Clinical Counterexample

Christmas Eve was but a day or so away when Jason Papaioannou, a young thoracic surgeon, received an urgent call to see an inpatient at Holy Wisdom Medical Center, a private hospital located in an affluent suburb on the outskirts of a major Greek city. Jason had recently returned home to Greece after completing his specialist-training in England. This private patient's case would be the young surgeon's first, so he was naturally thrilled by the opportunity. Elias Tsoukatos, a prominent pulmonologist, had requested that the patient undergo an immediate surgical biopsy.

As excited as Jason was over his first case, he couldn't understand why this relatively routine procedure seemed to be treated as a pressing emergency. Especially with Christmas Eve just around the corner, it seemed odd that the biopsy couldn't be scheduled for sometime soon after the holiday.

When Jason arrived at the hospital, the head nurse dashed across the ward's corridor to greet him. "Dr. Papaioannou," she said, "thank goodness you got here so quickly; your patient isn't doing well at all postoperatively. He developed a persistent fever, which has spiked to 103.8°F (39.9°C) despite antipyretic treatment. And after three transfusions of whole blood, his hemoglobin remains low…as low as 7 g/dL."

Utterly bewildered by what he heard, Jason said, "I don't understand; I've never operated on Dr. Tsoukatos's patient, nor have I even examined him…ever!" She quickly responded that Dr. Tsoukatos had seen to it that he, Jason Papaioannou, was identified as "the attending physician" in the official hospital records. "Please take me to the patient at once," the young surgeon said, astonished to learn that he was handed clinical responsibility for a patient he had never even met!

In a luxury suite with drawn blinds and very little ambient light available, the patient was lying in near darkness, yet it was still plain to see he was clearly exhausted and as pale as the white linen sheets that covered him because of his anemia. The man appeared moribund. He was burning up with fever and violently shivering with chills, his breath came with great effort, and he clearly suffered a great deal of pain. The patient was unable to walk due to pathologic fractures present in the right femur and left tibia secondary to bony metastases. Blood-borne, generalized dissemination of lung cancer was present in remote sites. The primary tumor itself had grown so large that its center was necrotic; this triggered generalized septicemia.

It would have been miraculous for this patient to survive for a few more days. The unfortunate bed-bound man asked "Is it absolutely necessary for me to go under the knife, doctor? Do you think I'll withstand surgery and survive? I **don't** really have the courage to be operated on and, honestly, I would rather **not** go through it."

Suddenly the young surgeon understood that he was chosen to be a pawn in a scheme planned by Dr. Tsoukatos. He knew for certain the patient wouldn't survive long enough to undergo surgery. So, the duplicitous pulmonologist wanted the pointless *surgical biopsy to be performed as soon as possible, as it would be to his financial benefit.*

If the urgent arrangements succeeded in getting the patient into surgery at once, and the man managed to survive long enough into the procedure, then Dr. Tsoukatos would at least be eligible to collect his commission on surgeon's fees (for the unnecessary biopsy performed) and on the private patient's referral as well as the commission on the private hospital's bill.

The cunning pulmonologist conspired to designate the young surgeon, as "the attending" physician; hence, all responsibility (liability included) would be focused on Jason. Moreover, Dr. Tsoukatos was setting up Jason, whom he later planned to blame for being too young and inexperienced in case the frail patient died during or soon after the biopsy procedure. So, the entire lost-cause case would have played out without any direct involvement of Dr. Tsoukatos.

Even if the unfortunate patient survived long enough for a final histopathology report to be issued, any protocol of toxic chemotherapy would have absolutely been out of question because of his unfitness and moribund state. Furthermore, even if chemotherapy were administered (despite all contraindications based on unfitness and old age), there still wouldn't have been sufficient time for it to benefit the patient. Hence, the whole idea of referring this case for a surgical biopsy had been futile from the start, because it wouldn't offer any practical benefit to the patient whatsoever; and Dr. Tsoukatos was well aware of that. This was a clear case of a dishonest physician's premeditated, malicious attempt to exploit a wealthy moribund patient.

Thoroughly disgusted, Jason telephoned Dr. Tsoukatos and gave him a dressing down he'd never forget. Jason reminded him that the patient was unfit for any surgical procedure and emphasized the point by saying "the patient was unlikely to survive merely having his hair cut and beard shaved by a barber, let alone a thoracotomy!" The young surgeon transferred the patient's case back to Dr. Tsoukatos— who was the referring physician in the first place, after all—and then he stepped away. Since that incident, the two physicians have never again spoken to each other.

Of course, the young surgeon paid dearly for doing the right thing. He made a potent enemy of

Dr. Tsoukatos, who was an established figure in his field, a renowned pulmonologist who had made a name for himself among his colleagues. Dr. Tsoukatos never again referred any other cases to Jason, but in addition, he actively defamed, disparaged, and discredited him for the rest of his professional life.

Continuation of Chapter 16

We all constantly endeavor to address the question of how much truth the patients can and should be told. One wonders whether or not an unfortunate human being can handle the whole, full, and absolute truth, especially in cases when it can bring about despair. In other words, should or shouldn't patients be informed when death is imminent?

Let me remind readers that this book was written to promote a broader viewpoint supporting patients' awareness of the truth about their case. Hence, I do believe that, at an absolute minimum, patients should definitely know when their diagnosis is cancer, no matter how difficult to treat or ominous their case or how advanced their stage really is. So, awareness of the diagnosis of cancer is non-negotiable in any case.

Of course, the truth is somewhat more pleasant and easier for everyone involved, if a patient's case happens to be one associated with a good chance of cure or with a similarly favorable prognosis. In that case one is happy to provide information honestly and in great depth; breaking news under such conditions is quite easy.

On the other hand, practical problems arise in the "Uncomfortable, Difficult Sessions" case addressed in chapter 13 (p. 129), when no reasonable chance for cure exist. In that chapter I described a way of gently talking to the patients regarding how they will be *"helped"* by "the treatment indicated" in their case. The part about providing information about therapeutic options has already been covered.

Patients usually don't ask too many questions, if they face a dismal prognosis, since they probably sense their doctor's uncomfortable situation. The patients subconsciously know the unfortunate truth by directly communicating with the doctor's subconscious. Still, what about the rarest cases, when ominous-prognosis–patients directly ask about elaborate details regarding their own stage, extension of the disease, their chances for cure, and the overall prognosis expected?

I still struggle over choosing the most appropriate way to answer that last question. I know that physicians are not—I repeat, not—allowed to lie to patients under any circumstances, let alone when they ask directly. Can concealing part of the truth be considered lying, though? To such unfortunate patients, one may indirectly—yet clearly—answer that their case happens to be…"difficult."

One may add that there's no guarantee whatsoever of complete success with the treatment about to be offered. If one says as much—precisely as one should—by truly feeling human compassion and with empathy for the patients, then the patients will subconsciously read the truth, they will sense it. And they won't continue to torment themselves by posing similarly prickly questions.

In my humble opinion, it would be inhuman and cruel for any attending physician to heartlessly utter words that absolutely rule out all hope in general to patients. I believe that such a cruel disclosure should be forbidden. After all, the whole idea of improving patients' quality of life lies with them getting to live as happy and comfortable as possible for the rest of their lives, if they can't be cured; this idea is totally incompatible with patients feeling adrift in an ocean of sadness, having abandoned all hope and feeling like death-row-convicts awaiting execution.

In other words, the doctors' obligation still stands, originating from age-old professional ethics: one must always attempt to provide some kind of palliation to one's patients, without resorting to lying, even if their prognosis is dismal. The latter is, of course, easier said than done; hence a physician usually needs some help toward this end from the patients' relatives and friends, by nursing staff, and by any other advocates involved. Some level of hope, regardless of how anemic, must always by instilled into the patients' soul; they should never be left in the absolute darkness of despair. They need even a mere glimmer of true light—the light of even a single candle is better than none. No room exists, however, for a fake candle used to deceive.

Now, let me proceed with what is a most formidably difficult question; What should one tell a moribund patient, whose death is *imminently* expected? Moreover, in that case, what can one do within the boundaries of medicolegal limits?

It would be inhuman to tell any human being that death is imminent, any moment now. It would be similarly inhuman to allow any patient to be left to the *agony* of impending death with maximal *anxiety*, facing death throes, death rattles, excruciating pain, and torment.

It is a given that medicine cannot always cure all diseases; it can, however, effectively and safely alleviate pain and suppress the pangs associated with imminent death. Hence, it would be *unforgivable* and cold hearted to abandon a cancer patient to torment and the anxiety that attends the moments immediately prior to death, since science is at least able to suppress that agony.

I was heartened to read a story published recently in BBC magazine* about effective steps taken to improve end-of-life care and promote palliative treatment and dignity in dying in Mongolia. Fifteen years ago, palliative care did not exist in that region. However, legislation was recently reviewed in Ulan Bator designed to prevent people from dying in agony. This was achieved thanks to the persistent lobbying efforts of a colleague there who persuaded her country's medical authorities and governing bodies that Mongolians deserve to die with dignity. It is hoped that more countries will follow the example set by Mongolia.

In other words, one never directly tells patients that their death is imminent. One instead tells them that they are experiencing a difficult phase and comforts them by encouraging them to be patient and to have courage. One doesn't have them undergo futile medical or surgical procedures. They shouldn't even undergo invasive laboratory tests or blood transfusions that will merely prolong patients' ordeals. We ensure that these patients are adequately hydrated (usually by intravenous infusions) and we make sure that sufficient doses of appropriate painkillers

---

* BBC News. Anu Anand's article: *"The woman helping Mongolians die with dignity,"* made public on June 21, 2017: http://www.bbc.com/news/magazine-40262012

are generously administered; the only appropriate painkillers for such patients are the ones that both suppress the agony of imminent death and effectively assuage the pain. I elaborate further on painkillers on the next chapter.

To summarize, in this chapter the viewpoint I expressed is that patients need to know as much of the truth as they can handle, without any excessive or elaborate details being disclosed that could result in unnecessary despair. Awareness of the cancer diagnosis is definitely a bare minimum requirement. Often, patients know their case is rather difficult to treat, without guaranteed outcomes, yet they also know that treatment will "help" them, when applied.

Under no circumstances are blatant lies allowed or unrealistic outcomes promised. We stand beside them by expressing deeply human emotions such as compassion, with empathy. If death is imminent, we refrain from torturing them with futile therapeutic maneuvers, and we actively care for them by offering palliation, peace, or even drug-induced euphoria, thus avoiding an inhuman death.

17.

Opiates – Painkillers and Other Medication

Clinical Counterexample

The renown surgeon Eric Fotas after completing a cholecystectomy (gallbladder resection) immediately filled out and signed his postoperative orders and handed the document to the staff nurse. The patient was to receive nothing by mouth, intravenous hydration, and perioperative prophylactic antibiotics were to be administered around the clock at specified intervals. In addition, he wrote "If the patient complains of any postop pain, 150 mg of paracetamol should be injected PRN" (PRN is a standard abbreviation for "as needed"). Paracetamol is the European name of a mild painkiller, known as acetaminophen in the United States (the main ingredient of Tylenol®, Apotel®, Panadol®, and similar medicines).

One of Eric's good friends, another surgeon who happened to be in the area and saw the postop orders, vehemently objected to his friend's instructions.

" What on earth do you mean by writing ' **If** the patient complains of pain ' ?! Can you possibly expect a patient might feel no pain whatsoever half an hour after having his abdomen surgically opened?! You can't possibly harbor so naïve an illusion. Of course, the patient will be in pain! I guarantee it! Thus, an effective regimen of regularly administered analgesic therapy will be required to control postop pain instead of the ' PRN only ' treatment you've prescribed, dear Eric! And with paracetamol, of all things! "

" What's more, do you really think a meagre dose of 150 mg of paracetamol will confer any meaningful level of pain relief after what this patient has just gone through?! Your patient is a fully grown man, weighing 209.44 lbs (95 kgs); a thousand milligrams of paracetamol might help if all he complained of was a headache, but he's just undergone an open cholecystectomy! You sliced through the skin, fat, and muscle tissue of this man's abdomen with a scalpel to get access to his gall *bladder. Surely you can imagine what that might feel like."*

Eric felt truly embarrassed; the dose he prescribed was wholly inadequate, but he was very uneasy about prescribing more potent, effective painkillers. He felt insecure and uncertain regarding specific dosages indicated, side effects, contraindications, etc. After all, Eric had received all his surgical training in rural Greek hospitals. He learned his specialty in an environment where he would have invariably and repeatedly heard a well-known cliché told with a shrug to postoperative patients all the time throughout Greece: " Hey…you've just had surgery! Of course, you're in pain. It's to be expected. Keep feeling it, but don't worry about anything. Everybody goes through it " * !

Pharmacology was taught during Eric's third year at medical school in Greek Universities. But after completing his formal studies, he never devoted any

---

* A shorter version of this cliché, translated into English, might be something like: "Hey, you're supposed to be in pain, since you've just been operated on!" In *Greek*, the cliché is: " ε, χειρουργημένος είσαι, θα πονάς…! " It is pronounced as: "eh, khirourghimenos ise, tha ponas…!"

time to review what he'd learned or attending continuing-education courses to update his knowledge of current opiates and how to administer them. He was under the false impression that only internists, anesthesiologists, and pain specialists needed to deal with that area of patient management. He had never ever taken a single course on analgesia during his six years of specialty training in surgery; nevertheless, he became a master at his craft—he was a gifted physician, widely considered a brilliant surgeon possessed of enviable skills.

<u>Continuation of Chapter 17</u>

Perhaps few readers will think it necessary to devote an entire chapter to pain management for cancer patients. But doubters will soon realize that pain management is a critical component of cancer care, and that medical communities in many countries, including Greece, do not pay sufficient attention to controlling pain and / or have a poor under-standing of how to use potent analgesics appropriately and to good effective.

Diseases, for a variety of reasons, follow diverse courses that lead to different outcomes in different patients, and that's certainly the case with cancer. As you now know, many patients can be cured or, with proper treatment, their disease can be controlled. Sadly, that isn't always the case; in some patients, disease progresses despite the best treatments medicine currently has to offer. When that happens, tumor cells can invade or impinge upon neuroanatomical structures and cause pain.

Fortunately, when cure or disease control isn't possible, we do at least have the ability to relieve any pain that might arise out of disease progression. We are equipped today with the means to alleviate pain fully and make patients as comfortable as possible. If physicians neglect to treat patients in pain when it is well within their capacity to do so, they are failing the most fundamental humanitarian tenets of their profession.

Strictly speaking, "analgesia" is the induced absence of sensibility to pain, and the drugs used to accomplish this are known collectively as "analgesics." In fact, analgesia can be induced by any number or combination of various modern medical techniques and methods, such as nerve blocks, epidural or even intrathecal administration of medicines, surgical or glycerol rhizotomy, rhizolysis, gangliolysis, etc. These are all available options that might be indicated or considered, depending on a patient's circumstances and whether they are candidates. However, the most commonly used method of treating pain in day-to-day clinical practice involves administration of pharmaceutical analgesics (or, colloquially, "painkillers").

Many categories of analgesics exist that possess different properties and vary in the effects they produce; some effects are desirable, while others are considered to be undesirable "side effects" of varying consequence and severity. Analgesics are grouped according to their chemical composition and their mechanism of action. Some, like aspirin, are well known and available over the counter. More potent agents include, broadly, narcotic (opioid) and non-narcotic (non-opioid) analgesics. Many different drugs are included under these two basic categories; they all have their rightful place in the therapeutic armamentarium and can be effective if used according to indications.

Yet, *just one* category of analgesics has proven *effective* for alleviating the most severe, excruciating pain patients suffer, as well as for *ameliorating the agony* that can precede imminent death. *Only opiates* are able to bring these patients the pain relief they deserve and we as physicians owe them that peace.

Opium has been with us a long time; humans have been harvesting opium poppies since prehistoric times. As for recent history, we don't read much these days about "opium extract," and few will remember "Sydenham's laudanum," and that this powerful narcotic preparation was freely available without prescription until the early 20th century. But their descendants are with us today, and we recognize names like *morphine*, pethidine, codeine, fentanyl, and similar contemporary derivatives. In addition, newer drugs such as tramadol have been synthesized and are available to us; these relatively newer opioids are considered much safer in terms of undesirable respiratory effects in comparison to, say, morphine.

Unfortunately, ridiculous, hysterical exaggerations have recently been published in favor of curbing legal opiate use and imposing further restrictions on approved indications for prescribing them, as well as decreasing their recommended dosages. Sadly, pain management has become politicized, and large international health organizations (such as the US Centers for Disease Control and Prevention) have taken it upon themselves to call for onerous prescribing restrictions, which makes no sense. One wonders, for example, how and when CDC, an agency created to explore and study ways to control and prevent the spread of *communicable* disease (e.g., malaria, tuberculosis, syphilis, AIDS, ebola virus, etc.) decided it is within their purview to tell physicians how they can and cannot treat their own patients. If illegal opiate abuse in communities has become a major public-health concern, that would logically seem to be a law-enforcement concern; it hardly makes sense to target patients who are legally prescribed these drugs under highly controlled conditions. It bears mentioning here that worldwide, recommended dosages of opiates have already been dramatically reduced during the past century.

In the 1920s–30s, morphine tartrate crystals were used in generous doses (each crystal contained the equivalent of either 30 or 60 milligrams) and doses could be repeated. Later on, smaller dosages of soluble morphine sulfate (which was easy to weigh, and doses could be individualized according to a given patient's needs) were used, as well as morphine hydrochloride (a single 20-mg dose could be repeated to a maximum 80 mg/day in 1948 *).

Interestingly, morphine is currently available for injection in 10-mg ampules. It is usually administered intravenously in smaller doses of 2–3 mg, which can be repeated, of course. Similarly, a dramatic decrease occurred in the "equianalgesic" dosages of codeine; in 1948, 75 mg could be given in a single dose up to 300 mg in 24 hours, while today the limit is down to 10–30 mg as a single dose with the total 24-hr dose not to exceed 60-90 mg of codeine phosphate. Similar reductions have taken place with all opiate analgesics.

I offer the following equianalgesic dosages below, for the convenience of all medical personnel authorized to administer opiates:

---

* V. Herzen, G Duhamel. Guide–Formulaire de Thérapeutique. 17th ed., J.–B. Baillière, Paris 1948.

- *Morphine* 10 mg *IM*: onset of action, 15–30 minutes; duration of action, 3–4 hours (after which repeat administration is often necessary)

- *Morphine* 30 mg *PO*: 30 mg; slower onset of action, longer duration of action

- *Dihydrocodeine* 60 mg: Note—this is indeed the equianalgesic dose, but it is *too* high, therefore it is NOT recommended; usually one administers no more than 30 mg of dihydrocodeine in a single dose (which can be repeated every 4–6 hours, as necessary)

- *Codeine phosphate* 120–180 mg *PO*: Note—this is indeed the oral equianalgesic dose, but it is *too* high, therefore it is NOT recommended; usually one administers 20, 30, or 60 mg in a single dose; one can repeat the administration of similar doses (taking care not to exceed a total of 240 mg in 24 hours)

- *Buprenorphine* 0.4 mg *sublingual*: Sublingual administration is considered superior to the use of injections, which can be painful; onset of action is slower—up to 3 hours—if given sublingually vs. injection, but the patients enjoy a longer duration of action, usually up to 6–

8 hours. (This analgesic is neither licensed for medicinal use nor available in Greece.)

- *Diamorphine* ("heroin") 5 mg *IM*: Medical use is not allowed in Greece or in most other countries, yet it is both licensed and available in *Scotland*; onset of action is 10–30 minutes after an intramuscular injection; duration of action, 3–4 hours. Heroin differs from morphine, because it does *not* cause nausea / vomiting; it can be useful for patients needing analgesia after a myocardial infarction.

- *Fentanyl* 0.2 mg (= 200 µg or "mcg"): It has an extremely short duration of action if given by injection (a few minutes usually, up to half an hour). Instead, one administers fentanyl via transdermal patches; transdermal administration avoids the inconvenience of injections altogether and offers cancer patients the longest-available duration of action; 72 hours per patch (or "TTS") applied. The onset of action after the first skin application can be as long as 18 hours, but there's no delayed onset with subsequent applications. The prolonged delay of onset warrants caution in order to avoid toxicity due to overdoses (no additional patches can be applied during the first

72 hrs after the first application). In addition to the convenience of transdermal administration vs. injection and length of duration of action, it is especially beneficial for patients unable to swallow (e.g., esophageal or gastric cancer etc.). More recently, this drug has become available for sublingual use.

- *Pethidine* 100 mg *IM*: Onset of action, 10–30 minutes; duration of action, 2–3 hours only, after which one needs to repeat a new dose to achieve adequate analgesia.

- *Tramadol* 150–225 mg *PO*: This is indeed the oral equianalgesic dose, but it is *too* high, therefore it is NOT recommended; usually one administers 50–100 mg in a single dose orally, which can be repeated taking care not to exceed a total dose of 400 mg in 24 hours. This analgesic is considered *safer* than conventional opiates due to fewer respiratory complications. Tramadol is also available in injectable form. It can cause elevation of transaminases in blood serum and other side effects.

I specifically refrained from mentioning intravenous administration of analgesics, to minimize any abuse of the information by persons addicted to drugs or attempting to gather information for nonprescription administration to cancer patients.

Unfortunately, in Greece and the world over, some colleagues have developed an aversion to the word "morphine;" the very sound of it seems to terrify them or carry a stigma. This fear is so extreme, I believe the condition qualifies as a genuine phobia. I'll call it *"morphinophobia."* Too many physicians seem to regard it as a "dirty" drug; they don't want to think about morphine, let alone prescribe it for inpatients who need it. This phobia is probably attributable to a lack of clinical familiarization or experience with opiate analgesics and / or an ignorance of proper dosing. I imagine in many cases these colleagues hadn't been adequately trained in how to administer the various opiates; hence, they dread causing respiratory failure or excessive sedation.

These irrational physicians have managed to infect a sizeable population of our nursing force in Greece with their own phobia. Many of our staff nurses require considerable encouragement to get over their fears, lengthy explanations about the need for these drugs, and additional training in order to get them to carry out signed orders regarding administration of morphine to inpatients.

Sometimes nursing staff rebel against administering morphine; they fear they would be held responsible for any unfortunate events, even if they followed protocol and meticulously administered the drug as prescribed by the physician. Sometimes they'll come up with schemes to avoid having to follow the orders, such as claiming they didn't administer the drug "because patients weren't in any pain at the scheduled administration times," despite the fact that this administration was ordered, not offered as a suggestion, or ordered PRN. When all other attempts to avoid giving morphine fail, the nursing staff just resort to the old cliché described earlier: "Hey…you've just had surgery! Of course you're in pain. It's to be expected. Keep feeling it, but don't worry about anything. Everybody goes through it."

This "morphinophobia" seems to have virulent properties, I'm afraid. It is even capable of crossing national borders and infecting so-called "medical thought leaders" who live in the theoretical worlds of government agencies. Agencies such as these are too-often populated by physicians who have forsaken medicine to practice government bureaucracy. No good can come of it, at least not for those who live in the real world. For example, recent CDC guidelines governing the use of opiates in cancer patients seek, yet again, to impose restrictions on dosages further and further, increasingly so as time goes by…on a world-wide scale. Fortunately, the CDC is a toothless organization in matters such as these. They can sit about in committees and cobble together all the guidelines they wish; they are unenforceable. Guidelines can be ignored, and they routinely are by the physicians who must care for real patients.

It is morally and ethically reprehensible to allow terminal-stage cancer patients to endure excruciating or intractable pain just because some careless, lazy, bored physicians didn't bother to study and memorize the opiate dosages, indications, and interactions during their medical undergraduate studies, and never bothered to keep current in pain management by pursuing continuing education after graduating. Such disgraceful behavior cannot be allowed to continue. Some physicians seem pathologically disingenuous; on one hand, they feign deep concern while stubbornly refusing to inform a patient they've been diagnosed with cancer (lest they cause any distress), yet on the other hand, they willfully abandon the same patient to experience intractable pain and die in needless agony!

Many papers in the medical literature have recently been published in favor of the medicinal use of *cannabis*. Such use is allowed—under specific terms and conditions— in some of the United States, including Alaska, California,

Colorado, Hawaii, Maine, Maryland, Michigan, Montana, Nevada, New Mexico, Oregon, Rhode Island, Vermont, and Washington. The reported benefits of cannabis include pain relief, reduced nausea and vomiting, appetite increase, decreased intraocular pressure (useful for treating some glaucoma cases), and euphoria. It has been well-documented in the literature that reasonable use of cannabis can significantly reduce the amount of opiates needed for analgesia in patients with cancer.

Cannabis, however, also possesses an undesirable effect: it could lead to addiction. Hence, this substance is specifically prohibited by law, or its use is highly regulated, in almost all countries of the world.

As this book is being written, considerable research is under way to explore the potential benefits of cannabis in cancer patients. For such research to succeed, all clinicians must reach a unanimous consensus on specific indications, contraindications, and dosages for this substance. If such a consensus could be reached, cannabis will likely play a role in improving quality of life in terminally ill patients by alleviating the anxiety, dread, and agonal moments that often precedes imminent death.

One important point needs to be clarified and emphasized at this point. This chapter urges physicians to use analgesics in adequate doses as appropriate and indicated for severe pain, but does *not* endorse under any circumstances deliberate overdose to expedite an expected death. Euthanasia is prohibited by law in most countries. More important, though, is that euthanasia has been prohibited for millennia by the Hippocratic Oath, which clearly states: " I will neither give a deadly drug to anybody who asked for it, nor will I make a suggestion to this effect " [*] OR: " I will give no deadly medicine to anyone if asked, nor suggest any such counsel " [†].

Our mission as physicians is to improve and extend human life. At the same time, we are duty bound to enhance or maintain quality of life by offering palliative treatment, at the very least, until the patient succumbs to their disease.

---

[*] Translated in 1943 from ancient Greek by Ludwig Edelstein, in Baltimore (Johns Hopkins Press, 1943). The original text in ancient Greek: "Οὐ δώσω δὲ οὐδὲ φάρμακον οὐδενὶ αἰτηθεὶς θανάσιμον οὐδὲ ὑφηγήσομαι συμβουλίην τοιήνδε"

[†] Translated in 1849 from ancient Greek by Francis Adams, as displayed in Encyclopedia Britannica.

Our obligation to help the patient ceases only when that life ends, but we must never provide the means to that end.

We promise our patients at the outset that we'll be there for them every step of the way through their treatment, that we'll do everything in our power to help them, and that help can come in many forms as circumstances demand. Therefore, it is imperative that adequate palliative care is provided...from the moment it becomes necessary to the patient's last breath. Anything less is a betrayal of our patients and makes a mockery of our integrity.

18.

Life Expectancy

Clinical Counterexample

I could scarcely believe my own eyes after reviewing Bob's chart. Bob was an indigent, homeless man who was transferred from a general hospital to the cardiothoracic center in Scotland where I was, at the time, completing my training as a specialist in thoracic surgery. Bob was specifically admitted to our facility because he had developed persistent hemoptysis (he was coughing up blood). While reading his case notes, I was astonished to find records documenting that Bob had been diagnosed with terminal-stage lung cancer 10 years prior to this admission. Moreover, pathology reports indicated that Bob had undifferentiated non–small-cell lung cancer (NSCLC). This is an ominous finding, as that histologic variant of lung cancer is one of the most aggressive forms of the disease.

I verified that the year of the first entries in Bob's case notes was indeed correct. I checked and double-checked dates on biopsy reports, CT reports, on correspondence, and on any and all dated documents in his file. All available evidence confirmed that, incredibly, Bob was diagnosed 10 years ago. The patient's condition at the time was objectively assessed as so dismal that he was treated with only a single dose of "palliative" radiotherapy administered in one session. This is a striking departure from the radiotherapy regimens patients like Bob typically undergo, which is delivered in fractions over multiple sessions until a cumulative total dose is received. For example, a radiation oncologist might determine that the optimal dose for a given patient like Bob would be 60 Gy administered 2 Gy at a time in 30 sessions over a period of six weeks (2 Gy × 30 sessions = 60 Gy).

Bob's physicians at the time of his diagnosis yielded to his persistent questions about how much time he had left to live. Bob was told that statistics show an average survival of up to eight months for patients with the same disease stage and cell type that he had.

Unfortunately, Bob took the statistical average as an absolute and firmly believed he would be dead in eight months. With the end so near, he decided he would live it up while he could. Abandoning all restraint, he lived as he saw fit, gave in to his hedonistic instincts, and embarked on an eight-month pursuit of pleasure and earthly delights. He quit his job, divorced his wife, sold his house, withdrew all his savings, and retreated to a remote, exotic, tourists' paradise.

Nine months later, Bob was all but broke. He had barely enough money to return to Glasgow, where he was no longer able to find work or put a roof over his head. He was reduced to begging in the streets for spare change and sleeping under a tattered old blanket and pieces of cardboard. There was no end to his misery. The many years of survival miraculously bequeathed to him were spent in wretched desolation.

Bob succumbed to his illness a few days after his last admission to the Scottish hospital—ten years after the initial diagnosis. Instead of the eight months he expected, Bob had inexplicably survived for another decade, as a homeless beggar.

Continuation of Chapter 18

Under no circumstances whatsoever should an attending physician predict or estimate life expectancy for any given patient. A humane, prudent physician should know better than to forecast what cannot be known with certainty. As Bob's story demonstrates, no matter how passionately a desperate patient pleads or begs to know how much time they have left, the physician must not cave in to such pressure and speak of statistical observations and theoretical survival times.

This is *not* to suggest that in such circumstances hiding or concealing the truth is acceptable. On the contrary, the entire premise of this book holds that all patients have the right to know the truths about their conditions; i.e., facts that can be demonstrated objectively using proven scientific means. If the diagnosis of a cancer has been proven histologically, we are obliged to tell the patient, because that knowledge is a proven fact free of any degree of uncertainty. We are duty-bound to disclose information we know to be true, certain, and unassailable.

Yet, no reliable scientific method exists that permits us to predict with absolute certainty *one specific* patient's life expectancy in any given clinical context. Indeed, enormous databases exist that permit statisticians to calculate average survival times among subsets of cancer patients with similar disease characteristics. But the results of these sophisticated calculations reveal little more than average values for discrete *populations*, which are end points of interest in studies, but they have no predictive value whatsoever for *one given* patient's survival.

In a population including a hundred patients identical to Bob, as far as specific sub-stage and histologic type, the statistical average survival might indeed have been eight months when Bob was diagnosed. Some sixty of those hundred patients might have survived eight months, yet there is no way to determine exactly who those 60 patients are going to be. Among the other 40 patients in that study, some survived much longer than 8 months, while others survived a much shorter time. Bob was lucky to have lived for ten years; but a similar patient named Alice died only nine days after diagnosis. The cause of death was an undetected "secondary deposit" in her brainstem*.

---

* Undetectable by CT scanning because the "deposit" was less than 3 mm in size. Computed tomography's "visibility of detail" is no better than 3 mm (this threshold is imposed by technical limitations due to blurring and visual noise as

The statistical average length of survival for the total population of 100 patients is indeed correctly reported as eight months, yet Alice didn't even have enough time to make out her last will and testament. Perhaps, like Bob, she had taken for granted that she would live for eight months, instead of the nine days she actually survived. I fear that every mistaken prediction or assumption can cause harm possibly comparable to that caused by the disease itself.

In a given patient's case the disease may progress at an unexpectedly rapid rate and cause death earlier than survival estimates suggest. Such a development would be especially tragic for that person. He won't be able to accomplish certain things he might have wanted to in the time he had left.

If a patient presumes he has eight months to live, he books an appointment with his lawyer, or priest, or he schedules a wedding date for his daughter so that he might get to see her married, and so on. If this person dies sooner than anticipated, obviously he wouldn't have accomplished those special things he considered personal priorities.

---

well as the need to limit radiation exposure to the patient). Thus, nodules, lesions, tumors (and pathologies, in general) smaller than 3 mm remain invisible to CT.

Moreover, the family of a patient who dies sooner than the statistics predict may suspect medical malpractice or some sort of error. This could lead to pointless legal proceedings that the plaintiffs can't win. Even if the courts find in their favor they can't resurrect the deceased. (And if they could, it would be a disservice to the formerly deceased, who would then have to go through the process of dying again.)

Unexpectedly, unfortunate outcomes can also come to be when patients survive much longer than estimated. In another case somewhat similar to Bob's, a daughter was struggling heroically to take care of her mother, who was suffering from leukemia. The daughter exhausted all types of leave she was entitled to (compassionate leave, unpaid leave, etc.) to remain beside her mother, never leaving her unattended, during the many decades that she unexpectedly survived. The daughter was eventually fired from her job. In time, she spent the last penny of her life's savings. Yet her mother still endured. The manner in which this case ended was so appalling and tragic it cannot, for decency's sake, be reported herein.

In conclusion, it is impossible for a physician to predict with meaningful precision *one patient's* life expectancy, even if the physician is familiar with the average survival of a *population* of cancer patients, as reported in medical literature. Patient survival data form a bell-shaped curve that represents a "normal distribution," as it is called in statistics. At each end of the curve one finds "outliers." Bob would have been an outlier at the higher end, while Alice would be an example of an outlier at the lower end of survival time. Neither was even close to the statistical average. Hence, no physician should provide important information, like life expectancy, that can't be determined with certainty. Moreover, providing inaccurate information can be expected to cause more harm than good. The patient is to be informed about all that is known, proven, *true, and accurate.* Informing about anything that fails to meet these standards is irresponsible, unprofessional, and benefits neither the patient nor the dignity of Medicine.

19.

For Physicians and Other Caregivers

Clinical Counterexample

Anthony Mekras was completely unaware that he had cancer. He hadn't been informed about his condition by anyone, either prior to or after he underwent surgery. At his family's suggestion, he had been seen as a private patient in the office of Mark Kalfadelas, a young surgeon recently returned to Greece from specialist-training abroad. The surgeon boasted openly and often of how "modern" he was and that he performed almost all procedures using "key-hole surgery," an informal term for video-assisted thoracoscopic surgery (VATS).

Similar to laparoscopic surgery, VATS involves the introduction of a miniature video (thoracoscopic) camera into the patient's chest via a small incision so the surgeon can view structures within the chest and the instruments used during the procedure, which are inserted through separate incisions. When VATS is feasible, it may offer some benefits over traditional, open thoracotomy.

Anthony couldn't have known, however, that Mark was in fact compelled to rely on this "modern" surgical technique—which involves external manipulation of long, fine instruments during procedures—because his hands were inordinately large, so large that it was difficult for him to attempt any open procedures involving the chest. It was this young surgeon's great misfortune to have been cursed with hands so enormous, they simply could not fit through a reasonable, medium-length incision into the chest cavity, as is required during thoracotomy.

The pretentious young surgeon's hollow boasting and self-styled claim to "modernity" were obnoxious affectations, but such effrontery paled in light of Mark's utter contempt for veracity and total indifference to patients' rights. Driven by selfishness, greed, and a grand sense of his own entitlement, he never deigned to tell his patients the truth when they were diagnosed with cancer. He justified this inexcusable behavior as a valuable time-saving measure; and to Mark, "time was money." Appointments were not to exceed 15 minutes, and the shorter the better. So, rather than risk spending extra time comforting shocked, newly diagnosed cancer patients sobbing in his office, he opted instead to avoid drawn-out, emotionally charged scenes altogether. Mark simply kept the news to himself and gladly allowed diagnosed patients to leave his office completely unaware that they had cancer. Once the unsuspecting patient left his office, another patient would be shown in, and so on, and so on. A steady volume of patients walking in and out of his office on or ahead of schedule meant a steady flow of fees to be collected for consultations, examinations, follow-up appointments, etc.

Keeping the consultations short—and patients unaware of their cancer diagnosis—ensured high throughput of patients examined and surgical procedures performed. He cared far more about the quantity of procedures performed than the quality of his work. He was a vain, ambitious young man who sought to establish a name for himself among peers and become so renowned a surgeon that he would have the longest waiting list of patients in Greece. This *he expected to accomplish all within a couple years of completing specialist-training.*

Mark was also jealous and power-hungry. He coveted the department director's post in his hospital. In a relentless, premeditated, subversive attempt to have the director fired, he undermined and berated the man little by little, day after day. Indeed, despite his youth and inexperience, Mark diligently conspired to displace the head of the department and, though woefully unqualified, assume the position himself as soon as the opportunity arose. He was the enemy within, a young upstart waiting impatiently to find some reason to lodge a formal complaint against the current director for any perceived infraction or wrongdoing that might be serious enough to launch formal administrative hearings or similar disciplinary proceedings.

One of the director's policies particularly infuriated Mark. He adamantly refused to sign discharge documents bearing a false diagnosis. At an absolute minimum, the director required that cancer patients at least be informed of the presence of "some cancer cells" when they were discharged from his department. Hence, Mark was forced, eventually, to inform Anthony that he had cancer. Unfortunately, he had never been keen on learning how to break bad news to patients, so he resorted to improvisation and telling half-truths. This sloppy, haphazard attempt to inform Anthony was certain to go poorly. And sure enough, upon hearing the news, the stunned patient dropped a glass of water onto the expensive carpet inside Mark's office, which further exacerbated an already messy situation.

Young Dr. Mark Kalfadelas set his teeth in rage; he was now more determined than ever to overthrow his director, as soon as possible and by any means necessary, so that he no longer had to waste his time informing patients of their diagnoses. Dealing with "hysterical" patients was beneath him; he didn't consider that his job. Mark was only interested in fame and fortune.

Legal Highlights

To some colleagues it may seem tempting to succumb to the easy solution of never disclosing a cancer diagnosis to their patients. By doing so, they avoid the unpleasant emotional burden, they have far fewer questions to answer, and they need not offer moral support to their patients. Also, consultation times remain brief, permitting them to examine more private patients in a given time period, and patients leave their offices looking calm...perhaps even smiling.

Such colleagues devise all sorts of pretexts and offer specious arguments to justify this practice, trying to make it appear "politically correct" under a humanitarian veil. According to them, patients have "the right to ignore their diagnosis" as much as to be aware of it; "patients should be spared from any distress or sadness" that might accompany knowing the truth. Other similarly ridiculous pretexts are often invoked or quoted to justify plain-old routine, deliberate nondisclosure.

A landowner can choose to ignore his property. When that owner is required to pay property taxes, however, as well as any outstanding fines imposed by town planning authorities and municipal councils, then he'll become very aware of his responsibilities. Ignoring his burdens or obligations will not make them go away. Similarly, patients will eventually become aware of their diagnosis (either accidentally or because of a potential progression of their disease). Hence, arguments in favor of systematically withholding diagnoses are ridiculous. It's all ploys and excuses. Myriad arguments have heretofore been listed and elaborated on this book that clearly demonstrate that patients have the right to know their diagnoses.

In the past, medical ethics were based on two-and-a-half millennia old texts: Hippocratic ethics and the Hippocratic oath. The latter, however, were not legally binding. So, there has always been some room for highly subjective or even biased interpretations. This is no longer the case. Most developed countries in the world implemented laws of their own in accordance with recently established principles set down during international conventions or based on declarations set forth by prestigious international organizations.

The United Nations Educational Scientific and Cultural Organization (UNESCO) held a General Conference in October 2005 in Paris and enacted the "Universal Declaration on Bioethics and Human Rights." In Article 3, Paragraph 2 of this declaration it is clearly stated that "The interests and welfare of the individual should have priority over the sole interest of science or society." Thus, the Hippocratic principle of the patient's primacy above all else is reinstated and ratified.

In Article 6, Paragraph 1 the Declaration states that "Any preventive, diagnostic, and therapeutic medical intervention is only to be carried out with the prior free and informed consent of the person concerned, based on adequate information," thus a legal requirement is born.

Finally, in Article 18, Paragraph 1 of the UNESCO declaration it is stated that "Professionalism, honesty, integrity and transparency in decision-making should be promoted, in particular declarations of all conflicts of interest and appropriate sharing of knowledge."

Similarly, the Council of Europe in 1997 enacted the "Convention for the Protection of Human Rights and Dignity of the Human Being with regard to the Application of Biology and Medicine." The legally binding (for all EU member states, at least) international text clearly states the primacy of the human being, prevailing over the interests of science or society (Article 2 of the EU Convention). It also necessitates obtaining "free and informed consent" prior to any intervention (Article 5). The EU Convention protects the patients' right to know any information collected about their health (Article 10).

The above-mentioned legal texts (The UNESCO Declaration and the Convention of the European Council) compel member states to take appropriate legislative measures to give effect to the principles set out. So, it comes as no surprise that almost all countries have laws protecting the patients' right to be aware of their own diagnosis. For instance, in Greece the Act 3418 / 2005 regulated the matters related to these rights of patients in Articles 11, 12 (¶ 2), 13 (¶ 4) as well as articles 2 (¶ 4) and 8 (¶ 2). Of course, similar laws exist in the United States, the United Kingdom, Australia, New Zealand, Germany, Japan, France, and elsewhere.

The importance of the existence of laws safeguarding patients' rights lies in that, nowadays, any potential breach of the law is considered a "criminal offense," punishable by courts of law. On the contrary, if it were merely a "violation of ethics principles" that a physician was accused of, then he / she would only face disciplinary "hearings" within a governing medical association or council, usually with limited disciplinary powers; temporary suspension of a physician's license may ensue from a disciplinary hearing (or even a permanent suspension).

Imposing a prison sentence, however, is an altogether different realm of punishment, which only courts of law can impose.

In many states' laws (for instance, in Article 12, ¶ 2 of the Greek law mentioned above), it is stated that patients' free consent should not be a result of misunderstanding, deceit, or threat. It is a criminal offense for a physician to threaten patients (e.g., using psychological coercion or creating a false impression of urgency) to obtain consent. It is inappropriate to create an illusion of "urgency" for undergoing same-day surgery or early morning following-day surgery by threatening "if you don't consent immediately, then your cancer will have metastasized by (the day after) tomorrow and, consequently, you'll die."

Patients are entitled to take their time (a reasonable length of time, that is) in order to weigh the pros and cons related to their decision; that is, whether or not to provide consent. A week's time might be considered reasonable for patients deciding whether to provide consent for surgery such as amputations and organ resections. Within the British National Health Service ("NHS") a month and a half (1½) is usually the maximal amount of time allowed for scheduling curative surgery after the date this patient was seen by the surgeon for the first time. If a physician considers the 45 days too long, one can seek a compromise time interval in the order of magnitude within the one- to three- weeks' range, so that extremes are avoided.

During these weeks, patients have the luxury of enough time to calmly think and weigh options, or to even seek a second opinion before making their decision. Of course, there should be an exception for emergencies, provided the emergency is well founded (e.g., hemoptysis or other hemorrhage, life-threatening bowel obstruction, and similar conditions).

The patients' clearly expressed consent is necessary for revocation of confidentiality, so that other parties be informed; e.g., family members, other relatives, or friends. No physician is legally entitled to inform relatives before the patient is informed (equally, no physician is legally entitled to inform only the relatives). To be able to inform relatives (or whomever), the prior explicit permission of the patient involved is required (Article 13 ¶ 4 of the Greek law mentioned above).

Research

We have no right whatsoever to present and propose any treatments as being "established" if those treatments haven't yet been unanimously accepted as effective and safe by all clinicians. Ambiguity is prohibited, because it could be considered deliberate and intentional. We are not allowed to suppress or conceal the experimental nature of any protocol still being tested by coercing patients.

Of course, it would be considered pure blackmail to force patients to enroll in experimental treatment "protocols" without them knowing the experimental nature of those studies. Rather than go untreated at all, patients may feel compelled by anxiety to sign anything, so they'll be treated one way or another, especially if they are unable to afford the treatment costs in poor countries in Africa, in Greece, and elsewhere. They may sign any uninformed consent lest they be deprived of some "miraculous new medication" too expensive for them to afford. They may elect to sign consent forms because of feeling indebted to the provider of the expensive medicines, even if they are unaware of their own exploitation as human guinea pigs. If unaware patients are told that they will be given new, expensive, purportedly established medicines—unavailable or unaffordable by their insurance—thanks to a tested protocol, then any consent forms signed by them are void.

No physician should urge patients to sign an ostensibly "routine consent form" in order to benefit by being enrolled into group X or Y that will receive some expensive medications, if it's all about an experimental protocol of administering the X or Y therapy. Any experimental or research nature of therapies proposed must be clearly explained as such to patients in plain words, in language they'll understand. We have the explicit duty to let patients know whenever we recommend an experimental, promising treatment whose efficacy and safety are still to be proven.

If a physician conceals the experimental nature of a recommended treatment, then that physician is exposed as a shameless, unethical scientist, a person who deceives weak, apprehensive, suffering patients for his own benefit, in the hope of publishing a paper with the subsequent acquisition of a research title.

No responsible humanitarian and serious researcher would want to be exposed as a fraud. Although that's precisely the risk he runs if he strives to recruit more and more patients who are not explicitly and clearly informed about being part of an experimental protocol, just to recruit a sample large enough to demonstrate statistical significance.

Such a researcher might also be suspected of possessing base motives; ample rumors have circulated about supposed bonuses and kickbacks paid under the table by the pharmaceutical industry for increasing the consumption of costly chemotherapy or anticancer medicines. Such astronomical costs can only be justified and billed to insured patients' clinical care if the costs are associated with proven effectiveness and safety.

Difficulties for the Attending Physician

The attending physicians are required to inform their patients in an appropriate way. One can easily fathom how difficult this responsibility is for physicians; one can also sympathize with physicians because of the difficulty of the task. Physicians need to be properly trained on how to break bad news to patients through appropriate courses or special curricula. Physicians also need to devote valuable clinical time to support their patients fully and provide answers immediately after the initial disclosure.

The physicians' duty to inform is also difficult because of the level of patience and benevolence demanded when the occasional patient happens to act out physically, possibly damaging furniture or other objects found in physicians' offices. Some patients may rapidly move from Denial to Aggression (please see the five stages of mourning and grief, in chapt. 6, p. 56), letting off some steam and venting negative energy.

Finally, delivering the diagnosis is difficult for attending physicians because the ongoing routine of breaking bad news wears them down emotionally; for every new case, attending physicians have to repeat anew all that's involved in declaring their participation in sharing the patient's sadness…with humanity and compassion.

Physicians, of course, are first and foremost human beings, vulnerable to the same diseases as patients, they personally understand what it is to mourn, and are subject to intensely deep passions and emotions—just like anyone else. Consequently, some aren't expected to endure functioning in the most difficult of clinical circumstances. Colleagues in some medical specialties that carry a graver burden than others may themselves be at risk psychologically after repeatedly having to break unpleasant diagnoses to patients. If a physician succumbs to a depressive disorder, in which case he can no longer properly and appropriately inform patients, then he must either ask for an expert's (e.g., psychiatrist's) assistance or suspend clinical responsibility for cases under his specialty. The physician can attempt to change to a less stressful specialty or leave medicine altogether.

One can opt for any of the above-mentioned alternatives if one cannot cope with difficulties of disclosure, though it is not recommended for one to resort to the easy solution of neglecting one's duty to inform; if one does so, then one greatly harms both one's own patients as well as the medical profession collectively by exposing its professionals, as a whole, to public excoriation.

Respect Patients' Right to Refusal

We need to learn to respect the patients' right to refuse any treatment recommended. If patients have been fully informed about their diagnosis and the consequences of refusing treatment, and if they are legally sane, then it is their right to refuse treatment on their own responsibility.

Results of some studies on patient attitudes have been published in newspapers (such as the British Daily Mail, dated May 30, 2014*): most physicians who were terminally ill would avoid aggressive treatments such as chemotherapy, and 88% of them would even choose 'do not resuscitate' (DNR) orders in case of a terminal event. They would much prefer to die in the comfort of familiar surroundings among their loved ones, rather than in a cold, impersonal hospital, looked after by strangers. No one can claim that the ill doctors weren't sufficiently aware of the consequences of their decisions. Every patient equally has the right to refuse, provided they've been fully informed.

---

* www.dailymail.co.uk/health/article-2643751/Most-doctors-terminally-ill-AVOID-aggressive-treatments-chemotherapy-despite-recommending-patients.html

In the past, it was considered appropriate to coerce some patients to consent to treatments because those patients were left utterly unaware of their true diagnosis, the course of their disease, and the consequences had it gone untreated. Those physicians from that bygone era who coerced consent were themselves under the illusion that it was both their right and duty to do so, for the benefit of the sick, who were, alas, steeped in ignorance owing to deceit.

Relatively recent history has informed us of the gruesome brutalities humans are prepared to inflict on their fellow man whenever the patients' sacred and ancient rights are violated. An extreme example of how bad things can get would be the evils perpetrated on prisoners in Nazi concentration camps during WW II who were subjected to bizarre experiments as human guinea pigs under the approving eye of the Gestapo. Today, no medical practitioner would care to be likened to the inhuman, monstrous atrocities of World War II. Thus, the principles of medical ethics make it imperative for us to respect and honor the legally sane, fully informed patients' right to refuse treatment, every bit as much as their right to consent.

<u>Consistency in Dealing with Patients</u>

Fellow physicians from around the world, proud of their superb training abroad, have indeed mastered novel, innovative, cutting-edge techniques; they are able to perform liver transplants, robotic surgery, and so on. In developed foreign countries where they trained, they had the opportunity to experience clinical-practice environments where all patients, without exception, had been fully informed about their condition and possessed a deep awareness of their cancer diagnosis. These young physicians became accustomed to health-care systems that consistently functioned with the precision of a Swiss watch; in other words, a system characterized by flawless coordination and synchronization of its multiple parts.

When these young physicians return to their own, perhaps poorer or under-developed countries, they shouldn't employ the single highly profitable technique they mastered abroad and pretend to have forgotten all they learned about the importance of consistently dealing with patients honestly and keeping them well informed. That is, it would be a shame if young colleagues didn't apply the entirety of what they experienced in clinical practice abroad—including what they learned about honestly informing cancer patients—when they return to their home country. If these young physicians don't actively contribute to improving clinical practices in under-developed countries, how can any progress in health-care practices be expected?

<u>Ways to Demonstrate Care and Affection for Patients</u>

All too often, physicians hypocritically state publicly that they vehemently oppose disclosing cancer diagnoses to their patients out of a professed love and care for them, lest they cause them any distress. There are, however, *far better* ways to express our caring affection:

1. We must accelerate the time it takes to establish histopathology diagnosis and determine stage; diagnosing and staging are reported as taking far too long in Greece (and elsewhere). When a suspicious-looking shadow is found in the lung on a patient's chest x-ray, then all subsequent appointments should be scheduled promptly, such as CT scanning and bronchoscopy. If we truly care for patients, we never deliberately delay bronchoscopy appointments in order to exaggerate the nature and complexity of the procedure and the level of expertise required to perform it as a means of convincing anxious patients that the costs involved are understandably higher than would be considered for normal or simple routine endoscopy.

a. After a shadow was detected on x-ray in the lung of one unfortunate patient, it took 40 days before he underwent chest CT scanning, after which he would wait another month and a half before undergoing bronchoscopy, and still another month after that before the histopathology report was available. Staging tests (brain and abdominal CT, bone scanning) were requested in accordance with "lab-test request practices" mandated by the patient's insurance company; ultimately, these staging tests were scheduled a whole month after they were formally requested. The patient was eventually referred for surgery a full six whole months after the abnormal finding on x-ray.

b. Another patient was finally referred for treatment of his lung cancer three years after an incidental radiologic abnormality was found.

2. When patients have already been admitted into a hospital, we inform them about their cancer diagnosis relatively early during their stay, if we truly care for them. By doing so, the newly informed patients benefit from being continuously under

observation and supported by competent hospital staff throughout the early, most upsetting phases of grief and mourning, as already described in chapter 6 (p. 56). Thus, the patients have time to overcome, to some extent, the initial distress and learn to cope all the while under constant care. They're much improved psychologically by the time of discharge; these patients are happy to be going home and are prepared to fight their disease. If we truly care for our patients, we don't withhold the diagnosis until they are about to be discharged. Sending them home immediately after hearing such devastating news would terrify them and deprive them of the benefits of in-hospital emotional support.

3. We only administer those therapies that are medically "indicated," if we genuinely care for our patients. We never subject our patients to procedures that are futile in their circumstances, just to bill for "expert services provided."

4. To elaborate further the above-mentioned point; we don't try to turn the desperate hopes of advanced-stage patients into profit by promoting costly extravagant procedures or major surgery

contraindicated in their case—not if we honestly do care for our patients.

Genuine Loving Care for Humanity

Physicians' personal encounters with cancer are very emotional. And, of course, physicians are not immune to cancer; many have lived with this diagnosis and have unadulterated first-hand experience of being patients themselves. Whenever physicians' stories of personal battles with cancer are published* †, they invariably affirm that *empathy* from all caregivers is critical to supporting patients as they endure the stress and strain of having cancer and undergoing treatment.

Empathy is defined as the direct identification with, understanding of, and vicarious experience of another person's situation, feelings and motives; in plain words, empathy is when physicians' actions speak of how deeply they care for their patients and how they're emotionally

---

* "Dr. Potarazu: The Waiting game: a physician's personal encounter with cancer." Dr. Sreedhar Potarazu's article, published on Fox News on May 4, 2016. Direct link for the article: http://www.foxnews.com/opinion/2016/05/04/dr-potarazu-waiting-game-physicians-personal-encounter-with-cancer.html

† Paul Kalanithi. When Breath Becomes Air. ISBN 9781473523494. Vintage ed., London 2016

invested in promoting their patients' psychological well-being.

It bears stating again that even in this day and age, some physicians still insist on withholding a cancer diagnosis from their patients to "avoid upsetting them" with unpleasant diagnoses. These colleagues ought to stop pretending and inventing pretexts out of convenience, simply to save themselves time and effort and start expressing true empathy by supporting, comforting, and answering their patients' questions. If they are genuinely that motivated by compassion, they will find the time to express it.

Finally, a number of major steps ought to be taken immediately to streamline care for advanced-stage or poor-prognosis patient care wherever legislative regulations regarding medical decision-making and medical conduct at the end of human life are lacking. This action is absolutely mandatory if our promises to newly diagnosed patients are to be fulfilled. As readers may recall, in difficult cases involving patients with an ominous prognosis, we promise that our medicines and treatments will "help" them; at present, medicine can only help terminal cases by offering sufficient pain relief and by using supportive care to make patients as comfortable as possible when death is imminent. Lack of regulations governing such care may lead to unfathomable consequences, as described earlier; for instance, the heartbreak of "successful" cardiopulmonary resuscitation of moribund patients who are "jolted" back to life, only to resume dying.

Thus, a desperate need exists for humane physicians the world over to lobby for the institution of global principles regarding the provision of relief in terminal-stage cancer care. "Macmillan Cancer Support" is a nonprofit organization of volunteers and other individuals in the United Kingdom that serves as a shining beacon illuminating the correct path. Similar organizations exist in Greece, such as the "Jane Karezi" and the "Galilee" foundations, and elsewhere. I do believe that truly humanitarian principles for cancer patients' relief can be put to practice everywhere on the planet simply by being honest with patients and respecting their right to know the truth about their condition, which should be revealed as soon as possible and explained with sensitivity and tact.

Since we, physicians, promise relief and comfort to cancer patients, we ought to be cognizant of all necessary details regarding the dosages, indications, contraindications, and interactions of analgesics. Together we all ought to strive, each to the best of our ability, to have national legislation modernized and improved in favor of humane treatment. *Dysthanasia* shouldn't exist in the 21st century; it is unnecessary, indecent, inhuman, and indefensible.

Instead of resuscitating dying, end–stage cancer patients, we need to remember that another function of the physicians is to pronounce a person dead. In developed countries, that's what they do when a patient is at last at peace; resuscitation in such cases would be obviously futile, if not cruel.

Physicians have a duty to encourage patients who have been successfully cured of cancer to speak out about their experience. Spreading the word, from the mouths of actual patients, that cancer can indeed be cured is the best way to offer genuine hope to newly diagnosed patients. The power of *hope* is inspired when it is based on truth, not on deceit and failure to inform. And so, to readers all over the world, I offer the following entreaty:

Please come forth and take the wonderful news of your own cure to the public. In doing so, you have through the authority of your personal experience, the *power to "transfuse" hope!*

Acknowledgments

My most humble and sincere thanks to:

First and foremost, my editor and friend, *George A. Rossetti*[1], for his dedication, talent, creativity and wisdom. He enriched my English with style and helped me hone my arguments eloquently for publication outside Greece. This English edition of "The Right To The Truth" would have never been possible without his tireless efforts over countless days and nights. I am eternally in his debt.

Prof. Peter Goldstraw[2], whom I served under as Senior House Officer at the Royal Brompton hospital in London. He encouraged me to publish this book. I learned a great deal from the example Professor Goldstraw set and by listening to him carefully and observing his personal approach to honestly informing patients about their diagnoses. He is defined by his impeccably skillful, bold surgical technique, deep analytical reasoning and high ethical standards, especially in adamantly adhering to

Staging principles. However hard I strive to model myself on this gentleman, I feel it is an impossible task! I consider him a lifelong, highly respected mentor, who taught me "The Art," as Hippocrates referred to Medicine.

Prof. Christos Mantzoros [3] from Harvard Medical School for his kind interest in my book and for encouraging me to complete the English edition.

The numerous people who encouraged me to go ahead and publish my ideas in a book that will surely displease many in the medical establishment in countries with dysfunctional medical systems. Among those who supported me, I'm especially grateful to *my partner*—for patience while I was so absorbed in writing this book for so long—as well as my sister *Liana C. Papachristou* [4], *Elena C. Selioni* [5] and *Nicholas Gage* [6].

The many experts who so kindly and generously took time to answer my countless queries on:

- Psychiatric aspects: *Demetrius Kourbetis* [7].
- Legal matters: *Justice Demetrius Doukas* [8], *Justice Foteini Keladidou* (ret.), *Ioannis Antoniadis* [9], *Giorgos O. Vavatsioulas* [10] and *Matthew Reddy* [11].

Friends who helped me better translate some specific terms or idioms into English: *Prof. Constantine Koupis*[12], *Sotirios Keramidas*, *David W. Jones*[13], *Alison Winter–Wright*[14], and *Joseph Keary*[15].

Friends who helped me translate some of the book's parts into French: *Dina Hassioti*[16] and *Vassilaki Papanicolaou*[17].

Anastasios Kafchitsas[18] for assisting me in matters involving Computer Science technicalities pertaining to—and essential for—the electronic publication of this book.

Jordan F. McQueen for the nice photograph (uploaded by him on 12.17.2014 on unsplash.com) used for this book's cover.

---

1 Writer, Author, Editor; Executive Editor (Emeritus), Gastrointestinal Cancer Research; Former Associate Editorial Director, 'ONCOLOGY'; LinkedIn profile:
www.linkedin.com/in/george-a-rossetti-9b14a972/
2 Emeritus Professor of Thoracic Surgery, National Heart and Lung institute, Imperial College, London; Honorary Consultant in Thoracic Surgery, Royal Brompton Hospital; Past President, International Association for the Study of Lung Cancer.

3 Prof. Christos Mantzoros, MD, DSc, PhD h.c. mult: Professor of Medicine, Harvard Medical School; Editor–in–Chief, Metabolism, Clinical and Experimental, Boston, MA.

4 Professor of classics (ancient Greek and Roman language, literature and history) at the Senior High School at Kalampaka, Greece. A graduate of the School of Philosophy, University of Ioannina. Expert in classical philology.

5 Biologist. Holder of a Master of Sciences with honors in "Biology of Reproduction" from the University of Thessaly, Greece, School of Medicine. A graduate of the Department of Biology, University of Patras, Greece.

6 Writer and investigative reporter for The Wall Street Journal and The New York Times. Author of the best–selling Eleni (1983), A Place for Us (1989), Greek Fire: The Story of Maria Callas and Aristotle Onassis (2000) etc. Born Nikolaos Gatzoyiannis.

7 Consultant Psychiatrist, head of the Psychiatric Dept., "The 424" military hospital in Thessaloniki, Greece. Colonel, Hellenic Army Medical Corps.

8 Presiding Judge at the permanent standing Court–Martial sitting at Athens, Greece. Colonel.

9 CDRE Ioannis Antoniadis, HN (ret.). Economist, Labor Law specialist. Former President of the Alumni Association of Greek Military School of Combat Support Officers.

10 Attorney at Law in Athens, Greece. Holder of a Master of Laws (LL.M.) in Banking, Corporate, Finance and Securities Law from the University of Pennsylvania (UPenn) Law School. A graduate of the School of Law, Aristotle University in Thessaloniki, Greece (LL.B.).

11 Attorney at Law, handling a substantial medical malpractice case load in Chicago, Il. Holder of a Bachelor of Arts,

Psychology and Political Science of the University of Michigan. A graduate of Boston University School of Law.

12 College Professor in Welwyn Garden City, Herts, UK. Scientist, B.Sc., MBA.

13 Author and IRS–official, a Physics graduate from Central Missouri State University, living in Liberty, Mo

14 Consultant Surgeon and Aesthetic practitioner in Glasgow, Scotland

15 Chief Medical Technologist, Irwin Army Community Hospital, former Commander of US Army 388th Multifunctional Medical Battalion, living in Topeka, Kansas

16 Professor of French language and literature, living in Trikala, Greece. A graduate of the « Université Michel de Montaigne Bordeaux 3 », Bordeaux, France.

17 A holder of a « Doctorat de littérature française, francophone et comparée », from the « Université Michel de Montaigne Bordeaux 3 », Bordeaux, France.

18 Holder of a Master's degree with honors on "Networks, Communications, Systems Architecture" from Aristotle University in Thessaloniki, Greece, School of Computer Science. Graduate of Computer Science, Hellenic Open University in Patras, Greece.

About the author

I'm a thoracic surgeon and current Head of the Thoracic Surgery Department at the 424 Military Hospital in Greece. It's a position I've held since 1999.

My early years were spent in my hometown, Kalampaka, which lies under Meteora, a picturesque rocky complex with post-Byzantine monasteries built on top. I studied Medicine at Aristotle University, in Thessaloniki, Greece. I've been practicing Medicine since 1988.

I began my specialist–training initially in Athens, Greece, then continued in the United Kingdom cities of London, Glasgow and Belfast. I'm a former Regent of the European Society of Thoracic Surgeons for Greece (2005–2010). My areas of interest include lung cancer, bioethics, medical ethics, and medical documentation. Click on this link* for more details about my scientific and medical work. I serve as a Colonel in the Hellenic Army Medical Corps.

My inspiration for writing emerged from career milestones and other events in diverse geographical locations and cities in the UK, Greece, United States, France and elsewhere. My first three books were written and published in 2016, two in Greek and one in English: *www.papachristos.eu.*

In favor of coffee (lots of coffe), wire fox terriers, humanism, history, photography, design and reading.

---

* www.icp-med.gr/engl/scientific/

About the book / Synopsis

Should all patients be informed when they've been diagnosed with cancer? If the answer is "yes," Who should break the bad news to them? And How is such news best delivered? How much of the truth can a patient handle?

Patients' inalienable right to know the truth about their condition ought to be guaranteed the world over. Yet this right is routinely violated. In Greece, for example, cancer patients are frequently kept in the dark about their diagnosis. In fact, this right is routinely disregarded all over the globe with appalling consequences.

In "The Right To The Truth," the author—a thoracic surgeon—presents *Counterexamples* inspired by events observed during 33 years of clinical experience, and he addresses each with well-crafted *Arguments* in favor of the patients' Right to know :

- for Trust
- for Protection from predators who would exploit vulnerable patients
- for understanding that Sacrifices are sometimes required to achieve cure
- for acquiring well-founded Hope
- for Overcoming fear of the unknown

The book :

- offers advice *to family members of cancer patients*, as it is usually they who shoulder the burden of deciding whether or not to have their loved one informed.
- offers thought–provoking ideas for those who care for cancer patients. Physicians, nurses, psychologists, clergy, and *friends* are all urged to be truthful with patients; lying leads only to suffering.
- repudiates hypocritical arguments that claim withholding the truth from patients "spares them avoidable distress," when the exact opposite is true. The hypocrisy behind brazen deceit inevitably becomes a source of harm to the patient. Myriad unethical, even illegal, wrongdoings *are exposed* that they should be banned from clinical practice once and for all.—